The

CarbNite™

Solution

The
Physicist's
Guide To
Power Dieting

John Kiefer, BA, MS

www.CarbNite.com

ISBN 1-4196-1310-3

*To Drumwright,
who always hoped
I'd write a book.*

Acknowledgements

I'd like give the proper thanks to those who had such a profound influence on my attitudes and, consequently, helped shape this book. To Mike Hamlin, my 11th grade Calculus teacher: Thanks for showing me that it's OK if you don't know the answer straight-away, but you should at least try to figure it out. And to Bob Glidden, my 11th grade English teacher: You made me realize that being skilled in the Sciences is no excuse for being poor in the Language Arts.

A Letter From My Closest Friend, Nicole Morgan

Hey,

I know you asked for a testimonial but I really don't want to write one. I'm sure you would have wanted Drumwright to write your bio for you, but since that's not possible, I thought maybe I could do it for you. See what you think.

John Kiefer started his academic career in electrical engineering before deciding to pursue sports medicine. Always unpredictable, he instead ended up getting BA's in physics and mathematics at the same time—in only three years.

From there, he decided to try his hand at the next level of academic endeavor: graduate school in physics. That is where I met Kiefer (he prefers 'Kiefer' to his first name for some reason; I think it suits him better than 'John'). He had this strange humility about him that was intriguing. He always seemed to pass tests with high marks without much studying and attributed his performance to luck—lady luck must be his best friend because he did it time, after time. He didn't even study for our qualifying exams (four four-hour tests covering various branches of physics) claiming he was just going to fail them all. Of course, he passed all of them with flying colors. It wasn't a case of false humility; he simply holds himself to incredibly high standards.

Since I've known him, he's excelled at a wide-range of endeavors. As a few examples, he designed and helped build a human-solar powered hybrid vehicle that won a national race; within a couple of months of starting as a programmer, he took over development of legal software designed to streamline contract disputes; consulted for a technology development company; prepared for body-building and triathalon competitions and successfully trained others for the same; and for a year he even taught 9th grade algebra. Kiefer's skills range the gamut from theoretical physics to music to philosophy, but with all these diverse interests and activities, there's been one constant: his passion for the human body.

Kiefer has been interested in maximizing his athleticism since he was a teenager. He's experimented with his diet and trained his body for years, but when he began writing his book, I half-expected that something else new and more interesting would come up. I've known him for a long time and he thrives on new challenges. It seems I underestimated his passion for his work. Instead of becoming tired of the voluminous research, his enthusiasm grew as he pieced together the puzzle. His excitement became infectious.

The most amazing part of seeing this process unfold was hearing Kiefer become more and more dedicated to the cause of providing the truth to others. Remember those high standards? Kiefer worked feverishly to craft a book that was clear and engaging as well as scientifically valid. He agonized over layout, pictures, diagrams and even word choices. The result is a book that answers your questions— even those you don't even know you have yet—and that is also a pleasure to read. If you are at all interested in understanding your own body, read this book. Kiefer's done all the research (a Herculean amount of research citations alone!) and he puts everything into context. You'll understand what you are doing and why. More importantly, you will see results—I know I did!

Let me know if you can use it or what,

Nicole

Yes Nicole, I can definitely use it.

Contents

The Guide

Food Lists

Meal Plans

Recipes

Citations

Index

The Guide

Preface

We can all remember being pulled down into the pit-of-endless-promises by doctors, athletic trainers, nutritionists and even TV psychologists. We see our ideal bodies at the far edge of the chasm, but the "experts" assure us, if we only follow them to the bottom, we'll be able to climb the other side and capture the dream of a forever-slim figure. Reluctantly, we follow. During the descent, our hopes shatter as we realize: *there is no bottom.*

Instead of leading you down a bottomless pit, this books aims to bridge the gap between you and your ideal-self. Everything, from the Food Lists to the Menu Plans, is designed with this intent—even the text. Information presented here is precise, pithy and perhaps even a pleasure to read. But, most importantly, it provides the crucial framework needed to succeed and nothing more. So, although critical, discussions about general health and wellness or metabolic diseases are sparse. This book focuses on rapid, permanent fat loss. Increased health and wellness follow naturally. For those craving dizzyingly in-depth and up-to-date information about diet, disease, health, hormones, metabolism and food, visit *www.physicsnutrition.com*; you'll also find information on upcoming books in the series.

Now, building the bridge to success is one thing; convincing you to cross is another. To cross fearlessly, you need confidence in the quality of the structure. References to more than 1700 supporting research papers should give you assurance, despite the short, crisp treatment of several complex subjects. So if a statement sounds too incredible to believe, the reference marks on the inside margin direct you to the overwhelming evidence located in the Citations section. The references mean to enhance your journey, not distract your focus. Paragraph referencing like this, however, makes it difficult to know which papers support exactly which statements; line-by-line citations reside at *www.CarbNite.com*, if you're interested.

Finally, unlike many texts, the FAQs are real questions from real people and present material not covered or not covered with great detail in the main text. Be sure to skim through them.

Let's get started.

Beginning The Journey

We've All Been There

Nearly all of us have battled with our weight—some of us as early as our teens, but many more as we reach our 30's, 40's and beyond. We've used every new diet, adhering to every rule, trying to squeeze every last promise from the text. Daily menus are earnestly followed, we purchase exotic foods, adopt life-altering exercise programs and, perhaps most burdensome of all, buy every recommended supplement. The religious fervor of few monks can compare with the zeal of our dieting discipline.

We fly through the first few weeks fueled by the nearly instantaneous weight loss. Confidence rises, excitement takes hold and we press forward. But then everything comes to a screeching halt. Almost as quickly as we lost the initial weight, our progress stalls. We're no longer losing weight, the food choices are monotonous, we're feeling weak and drooling over decadent treats as if we haven't seen food in months. Believing we've done something wrong, we return to the pages of our current dieting bible and look for the missing details that can put us back on track.

But we're doing everything right. Calories are in the allowable range, there's not too much fat or too many carbs and we're getting plenty of exercise. What's wrong? Frustration replaces confidence then quickly turns to desperation. We cut calories. We ratchet up the exercise. We cut the fat. We cut out sugar. We cut out more fat. Still, little progress is made.

Disgruntled and disheartened, we finally throw up our hands and we quit. Clearly the diet didn't live up to the claims, but we normally blame ourselves for the disappointment. We figure we'll give it another try further down the road when we can devote more time, as if we didn't rearrange our entire lives and sacrifice precious time already. Even after we gain all the weight back, like brainwashed disciples we defend our diet of choice until the end, reciting, "It really worked for me." Our audience looks in disbelief at our overweight, out-of-shape body.

✧ ✧ ✧

Thousands of people experience this situation every year. Many popular diets are excellent for achieving health goals like lowering cholesterol and triglyceride levels or managing conditions like insulin resistance. Problems arise when using popular diets to achieve a goal for which they were never intended: fat loss. Manipulating the different aspects of the body responsible for fat loss, namely metabolism, hormones, fat cells and enzymes, defies conventional methods and requires a radically different approach than those intended for improving other aspects of health. Current dietary plans improve specific aspects of health and assist weight maintenance; the usefulness, however, ends there. Don't misunderstand: good health is always a concern. But if your goal is weight loss and, in particular, fat loss—cellulite, flabby butts, beer bellies and love handles—then you've been using the wrong tools.

The Puzzle

Unlike many in this field, I'm not a medical doctor or nutritionist to the stars: I'm a physicist. Like you, spending years trying to conquer my problem with body fat left me tired and frustrated. I've tried every diet imaginable—low-calorie, low-fat, low-carb, high-protein, zones, phases and many more—while attempting to erase the stigma that first began when, in the middle of my sixth grade class, another student looked me square in the eyes and said, "You're fat."

In the following years, firmly committing to weight loss was no small task. The late 80s witnessed a flood of discoveries about hormones, food, metabolism and fat cells that overwhelmed experts in the fields of health, nutrition and weight loss. Faced with a million scattered puzzle pieces, all from the same box, experts began arranging pieces to form their own images. There was only one problem: nobody knew what the final picture should look like.

Beginning with relatively few, nicely fitting pieces, they continued by expanding to broader and broader topics. As pressure mounted to explain the growing number of discoveries, interpreting study results liberally and often incorrectly became commonplace—pieces that didn't quite fit were beaten into place. Rather than clear, crisp images, these randomly created mosaics fueled an eruption of new and speculative diets. Unfortunately, the mosaics contained gaping holes and incorporated only a small fraction of the pieces.

The surge of research and speculation did, fortunately, set a renaissance of sorts into motion. Diet books, with their new theories, needed support and authors began including citations. The diet industry renaissance coincided with my growing interest in weight loss. Living within minutes of an extensive medical library, my curiosity led me to examine the offered proof by consulting the original scientific papers.

I remember the weeks spent looking up, xeroxing and reading numerous journal articles. It took time to learn the terminology, but within months I'd made my first startling discovery: the research available, even some of the research cited, did not support one author's theory. The cites consisted primarily of nicely fitting studies along with a few results twisted beyond recognition—the obvious smashed-to-fit pieces. The author ignored or belittled everything else.

Insatiably I began checking the validity of other diets over the following years, accumulating vast stores of research in the process. I eventually abandoned the pseudo-scientific diet books and began seeking my own answers. I wanted to know why it seemed nearly impossible to lose my body fat and why so many others were having the same trouble. Was losing the extra pounds really hopeless? Or did some method of stripping fat from the body, something effective for *everyone*— not just the extremely obese—exist? If such a method did exist, I was going to find it and, well, if it didn't...at least I'd know enough to never get duped into trying another fad diet.

Being a physicist gave me a different perspective than most in the field of diet and weight loss. Relying on the research of others when pursuing your own work is essential to success in the academic world of physics. You can never assume any-thing if you expect to be successful. You need scientific proof. So I applied the same principle as I searched for a solution.

The mind-boggling amount of information and numerous considerations gave me the exact same million-piece-puzzle others had already grappled with and, still, no one had the slightest idea of the final picture. I refused to throw valid pieces away or distort results to my own ends. If only a quick glance at the answer was possible. After reading over 20,000 peer-reviewed research articles, a stroke of luck turned out to provide the badly needed glimpse of the completed picture. A single event helped pull together years of research and The Carb Nite Solution emerged.

Destined to Fail

The solution to all our problems rests in the design. All the diets you've tried were designed for one of two purposes. Nutritional plans intended to improve athletic performance hold the spot of oldest special-purpose diets. Low-fat diets started in this area as did another popular diet, The Zone. Whether they actually improve performance and what kind of athletic performance they improve—endurance, sprinting, strength, power—is the subject for another book. Both, however, wormed into the mainstream market as fat loss programs, an area where neither is well suited.

The second and most common purpose involves improving a condition known as Syndrome X. Syndrome X describes a collection of metabolic diseases such as insulin resistance, high blood pressure, high triglyceride levels, high LDL cholesterol levels, low HDL cholesterol levels and, the only visible symptom, central obesity. Plans target controlling and reversing aspects of Syndrome X one at a time. Some only target cholesterol levels, others insulin resistance and still others high blood pressure. Over the years tweaking these diets to tackle more and more aspects of Syndrome X led to less and less effectiveness. Stretching a plan beyond its original reach crippled the previous benefits. A recipe originally resolving one aspect of Syndrome X can't be expected to tackle every aspect, like obesity.

You don't need to imagine what happens when diets designed for different purposes offer the promise of fat loss because you already know. They rarely deliver. To some degree, they do reduce *weight,* but only as a side effect of their original intent. As many now suspect, little of the weight lost comes from body fat—the majority may just be stored water, carbohydrates and muscle. It's easy to see why so many different diets—low-carb, low-fat, The Zone, South Beach and others—perform identically when used for fat loss: the original design was never meant to produce fat loss at all. We need a tool created *specifically for fat loss,* not something with the side effect of weight loss.

The solution, the right tool, does exist. Unlike any previous diet, The Carb Nite Solution is designed specifically for ongoing fat loss—and I emphasize *fat loss,* not just weight loss and not just fat burning. For the entire time you're on the diet you will burn the stubborn body fat deposits on your thighs, waist, stomach, love handles, underarms and everywhere else. Every diet thus far has failed to accelerate the loss of body fat. Sure, some may help you to burn fat, but it's the fat you eat (dietary fat), not the fat you're trying to get rid of (in this case, body fat).

The Carb Nite Solution is a tool, not a lifestyle. Designing one diet to at once promote optimal health and rapidly shed body fat is nearly impossible for several reasons. Often, lifestyle diets promote specific health benefits and cause only a small amount of fat loss as a side effect. On the other hand, The Carb Nite Solution is focused on body fat loss. Fortunately, the

6

process of losing fat reverses Syndrome X. It simultaneously raises HDL cholesterol levels, improves insulin sensitivity, and lowers triglyceride and LDL levels. At the base of all these problems is excess body fat, so it's no surprise that deflating the spare tire improves many of the deadly features of Syndrome X.

The Road Ahead

Don't be fooled into thinking The Carb Nite Solution is just another Frankenstein creation that's worth a try. Welcome to the world of power-dieting. Food produces powerful, drug-like effects and as with any drug you need to know how it affects your mind and body. The Carb Nite Solution not only teaches you how to rid yourself of all the excess body fat but in the process you'll discover several things about yourself. You'll quickly learn how much extra water and carbohydrates your body normally stores and how long it takes to get rid of the surplus. You'll learn how to eat with convenience and ease, controlling hunger all day long. You'll learn exactly how common items like caffeine affect you. You'll learn how carbs can heat up the night while giving you a good night's sleep. In short, you'll learn exactly how your body reacts to things you normally don't think about twice.

Within a few days of starting the diet, you may discover some shocking things about your body. Though not a new experience for all, stripping the carbohydrates from your diet will produce profound changes; and removing carbs from your daily meal plans is exactly what you're going to do for the first nine and a half days. These are your first few *fat and protein* days. Water weight falls away. Bloating after a meal becomes

7

a distant memory. Some sluggishness may strike briefly, but a fresh sense of calm, cool collectedness quickly follows. Your mood stabilizes, your body lightens, and you realize you've hit your stride. You feel like you could do this forever.

But you don't need to. Actually, it's not that you don't need to, you can't. On the tenth night comes a treat. More than a treat, it's actually the key for fat loss success that's been lying dormant in the research for decades. It's Carb Nite™, the solution to all your past dieting frustrations—especially the frustrations of those controlling carbs.

The tenth day unfolds as a typical fat and protein morning, just as the previous nine days, but the thought of Carb Nite starts a small trickle of excitement, building into a torrent as the afternoon rolls around. You take note of pastries and pasta, chocolate and cheesecake, donuts and daiquiris. The temptations approach from every direction: Are you on the verge of stumbling, tantalized by all these decadent treats? No, you have a secret—you're seeking them out for your dieting pleasure. Yes, dieting pleasure. Carb Nite is about the treats and sweets because carbohydrates matter most. Rising insulin levels in response to all the sweet, sticky, crumbly carbs is the secret behind Carb Nite's magic. Anticipating this opportunity to feast and enjoy what seems like a break from the diet, you find yourself noticing all the things you've given up over the last nine and a half days. You're about to enjoy them all and you know it's a necessity. Your success depends on a full enjoyment of Carb Nite. What many consider a set back on any diet, a pleasure plagued with never-ending guilt, instead creates the hormonal afterglow essential for the success of this diet—the reason for calling The Carb Nite Solution a power-diet.

Carb Nite ends with a warm feeling all over. Your body's disabled ability to convert carbohydrates into fat causes the overload of carbs to be burned off as heat—this in addition to a spike in overall metabolism caused by the sudden shot of carbs. Weathering the rise in body temperature smoothly transitions to a good night's sleep. Sleep will be deeper and more sound than normal from an increase in your brain's 'feel good' hormone, serotonin. Again, the feel-good sensation is caused by the late-day carbs. You may even find yourself experiencing dreams more lucid than ever before. The only thing interrupting the night's sleep might be some muscle cramping if you fail to drink plenty of fluids and take other minor precautions.

The next morning, morning eleven, you awaken to…fat and protein. Carbs are a distant memory by noon and you feel yourself easing back into the groove. Not to worry, you won't suffer another nine-and-a-half-day stretch without carbs. For the week, the 30 gram daily limitation on carbs—the amount of carbs in two slices of white bread—is still in effect, but now you have a choice: What night to make Carb Nite. Maybe you have a dinner party Sunday night or a date night with the spouse on Friday or even a special celebration for one of the kids on Saturday. Whatever the occasion, or for no occasion at all, your once-a-week Carb Nite will be the night of your choosing—assuming you've given yourself enough time since your last Carb Nite.

And this is how it is for possibly up to six months. You routinely take a reprieve from the severe carbohydrate restrictions of the week to enjoy everything you've been missing—everything you've probably been missing for years. Carb Nite, once per week, in combination with severe carbohydrate restriction lays the groundwork for achieving the body you once had or always wanted.

Often Ignored Hazards

Muscle: What Are You Willing to Lose?

While sitting in the lobby of the restaurant waiting for your reservation, a child grabs your attention as he flexes his arm, mimicking the obvious gym rat walking by. You glance away to hide your thoughts: visibly defined muscles really do portray a sense of health, confidence, beauty and attractiveness. Nostalgia for those school days of a tight, toned figure well up inside. You can't wait for the opportunity to see yours take shape again.

✧✧✧

The essential goal for any weight loss plan should always be the preservation of muscle. Maintaining muscle size and strength during weight loss nearly guarantees the lost weight to come from water, carbohydrate stores and most importantly, body fat. Fat loss results when the focus shifts from simple weight loss to losing weight while saving muscle. Hence the reason for stressing fat loss throughout the book and not merely weight loss. The Carb Nite Solution is not a weight loss diet; The Carb Nite Solution is a fat loss program. An emphasis on sustaining muscle and consequently losing only body fat is still consistently ignored by other diet plans.

You may be wondering why the short sermon on insuring fat loss as opposed to weight loss. During an otherwise uneventful conversation with someone about popular diets, he volunteered a striking comment, "Who cares what kind of weight I lost?" There are three important reasons why everyone should care.

1) Losing body fat makes you healthier while losing the same weight as combination of fat and muscle actually degrades your health. In other words, by losing fat you can decrease your chances of developing disease. By losing the same amount of weight from a combination of muscle and fat, you increase your chances of developing disease.

2) Muscle tissue is an important, metabolically active tissue. By losing muscle tissue you reduce your metabolism and make it easier to regain the weight you lost.

3) Laboratory animals, subjected to calorie deprivation— either throughout life or during their final years—live longer than well-fed peers. Years of research on this phenomenon show the loss of strictly body fat, not muscle, explains the extended, active lifespan.

Are *you* willing to lose vigor and vitality? Or maybe you'd rather focus on losing those hips or love handles.

Fat Cells: A Formidable Enemy

It seemed too good to be true. The excitement from losing weight at such a fast pace was dizzying. Low and behold, it was too good to be true. You denied the symptoms, hiding the facts from yourself. Maybe you ignored it for a week or even two, but now a month has passed. You feel the phrase urging forth at every inquiry about your diet. You fight to hold back the mantra of defeat. On one lousy day you finally cave to reality by uttering the most dreadful phrase among dieters, "I've hit a plateau."

✧✧✧

A plateau, as applied to dieting, describes the situation normally occurring within the first few months of a typical weight reducing diet. No matter what you do, you simply cannot continue losing weight. All dieters on nearly all plans experience plateaus. Fat cells determine significantly when or if plateauing occurs.

As obvious as it may seem, fat cells store the fat in your body. They're not made of fat; they just hold it. Collecting in large amounts around the internal organs and under the skin, fat cells are like little balloons inflating as they fill with additional fat and, once full, signal the body to create many more. When body fat reserves dwindle, a large number of fat cells sit empty because fat cells rarely, if ever, die. Even fat cells responsible for your baby-fat—the fat everyone said was so cute while pinching your cheeks—still lurk beneath your skin. Not only are fat cells practically immortal, your body can create an unlimited number at any age.

There is an up side. Full fat cells give the body an intense message signaling the release of excess body fat stores—metabolism rises, hunger loses intensity and fat cells empty out while refusing to store more fat. This contrasts with the popular notion that obese and overweight people have slow metabolisms. In fact, being overweight raises metabolism and accelerates fat loss. In the beginning, the greater the amount of body fat to lose, the more quickly it's lost because all those extra fat cells overwhelm the body with a signal to waste energy. And why not be wasteful when there's plenty of energy in reserve? The massive amount of rapid weight loss is the exact reason diet book authors love to showcase the success of their diets using obese participants—they would be equally successful on any diet plan, at least initially.

But as helpful as bloated fat cells are to the dieting effort, empty fat cells are nothing less than catastrophic. Dieting alone normally causes debilitating metabolic changes within a few days and emptied fat cells intensify the signals. The body halts fat burning—both dietary and body fat—metabolism nose-dives and hunger grows uncontrollable. Eating even loses the ability to satisfy. The excess of empty fat cells tells the body it's time to refuel and without a proper plan, you're likely to oblige.

When popular diets bring you to this point, you experience a plateau. All diet plans create empty fat cells and risk plateaus. Current attempts at a solution are rash and crude, making the situation worse. Using these plans only offers the chance of emptying a few cells while failing to even ease this difficult task. Losing anything more than a few pounds of fat sounds bleak—your progress screeches to a halt before even coming close to your goal. The Carb Nite Solution finally gives you the power to tame the dreadful effects of these little cells, avoiding the anxiety and aggravation of another plateau.

Rebounding: A Dreadful Conclusion

Weight loss stalled and determination wavering, you choose relief to torture—dieting is abandoned, if only for now. As feared, you feel the weight creep back in less time than it was lost. The daily climb through the numbers on the scale suggests things aren't as bad as imagined. You lost 30 lbs and gained back 30 lbs, but something doesn't quite feel the same.

You can't explain the new sense of softness on your thighs and around your waist. You expected your energy to return with the weight; it didn't. You expected your strength to return; it didn't. You expected to look just as you did before; you don't. There's something going on. You check the scale again. There it is in black and white: you really do weigh the same as before. What's different?

✧✧✧

As difficult as losing weight may seem, current weight loss plans make regaining the pounds a breeze. This rebounding effect—gaining the weight back in a much shorter time than lost—is a natural consequence of traditional weight loss plans, mainly because of fat cells. But there is a second, much worse aspect to rebounding, one associated with stress.

Affecting more than just med school students and parents of unruly teens, stress plays a role among dieters as well. And, as anyone who's experienced dieting knows, trying to lose weight is psychologically taxing. The physical strain experienced by your body, however, normally escapes attention and the combination of these two—mental and physical—creates a state of constant distress.

No conversation involving stress is complete without a brief discussion of cortisol, levels of which rise in response to stress. Cortisol levels normally only increase at night and during exercise, situations resulting in increased body fat burning. These bursts of cortisol drop quickly upon waking or cessation of exercise; in contrast, levels remain elevated for long periods, sometimes days, in response to chronic stress. Connecting the dots reveals an unwelcome conclusion: typical dieting keeps cortisol levels elevated for the duration. Soaring cortisol levels bear a large amount of responsibility for the loss of muscle described earlier, but another, possibly worse result comes from this enduring elevation.

Being familiar with the world of nutrition through your experiences with dieting, you probably know that eating carbohydrates causes a release of insulin in the body. Nearly all weight-reducing diets cause substantial and often sustained insulin release along with stress. Normally, levels of only one—insulin or cortisol—are elevated at any given time. The simultaneous increase in insulin and cortisol levels causes a terrible problem, one you'll experience using these weight reducing diets: the creation of an abundance of new, empty fat cells. This does two things. First, it slows your fat loss progress more quickly, hurrying the advance to a plateau. Secondly, when you end the diet the newly created supply of empty fat cells help make you fatter than ever before.

Picture someone starting at 180 lbs, 30% of which is body fat. Having only briefly achieved their goal of reducing body weight to 140 lbs—possibly a wedding-day weight—the loss quickly returns. Returning to a former number on the scale doesn't sound so bad until experienced: it's like inheriting a different body. The regain no longer consists of a balance between muscle and fat, but is primarily fat. The loss of precious muscle combined with an appearance of the many new fat cells make the excess fat storage at a familiar body weight possible. Now, instead of being 180 lbs at 30% body fat, they're 180 lbs and 40% body fat. Being actually fatter than before starting the diet, they feel softer, less energetic and weaker.

The eventual regain of weight—over several years—holds fewer consequences than rebounding, but still carries a serious repercussion: an indefinitely slowed metabolism. For many, even escaping a short-term rebound does little to prevent this long-term gain. Regardless of timeframe, weight regain creates frustration among dieters echoed by health-care professionals when they ask: Why diet if you're only going to gain the weight back? Nearly eliminating the rebound effect and narrowing the possibility of long-term weight regain, The Carb Nite Solution renders the question meaningless. *Fat loss can be permanent.*

Problems With What We've Been Trying

Cutting Calories

You can't help but notice the methodical chanting of athletic trainers, nutritionists and even your friends who watch Oprah religiously: calories in, calories out. What does it mean? Sheepishly you ask and discover the simplistic logic. Lower caloric intake to less than daily needs and you're guaranteed the slim figure you've been imagining for years. You anxiously plan an 1800-calorie menu for the next day. A couple months of limited success pass, but you don't look or feel as good as you ought and the weight loss fades—you must be eating too much. You plan 1400-calorie menus and your march to slimness slows once again. Then 1200-calorie, 1000-calorie, 800-calorie menus fall like dominos as you struggle to sustain mental and physical energy. How long can the downward spiral continue? And why isn't a fitness model staring back from the mirror yet?

✧✧✧

The single most popular method of weight loss is cutting calories. Despite the popularity, the cutting calories approach carries many heavy costs. The first is muscle loss. How much muscle might you actually lose on the traditional low-calorie diet? In the first two months of low-calorie dieting about half the weight lost comes from lean tissue. That's one pound of muscle lost for every pound of fat lost. Over time this percentage drops to anywhere from 25% to 15%, meaning normal dieting continues to disintegrate muscle at the rate of one pound for every three to four pounds of fat.

Imagine setting the goal to lose 30 lbs of body fat. You begin by losing 20 lbs of total weight during the first two months. Concentrating solely on the number displayed by the bathroom scale, you're unaware of the loss of 10 lbs of muscle along with only 10 lbs of fat. Over the next two months you lose another 12 lbs but again, the total is not body fat—only 9 lbs came from fat. Four months have passed and the scale welcomes you with a pleasant surprise: 32 lbs vanished since beginning your diet. Unbeknownst to you, the scale masks the terrible truth that only 19 lbs of fat is gone with another 11 lbs to go if you want to reach your goal. The destruction of 13 lbs of lean mass also occurred. Scales often deceive us in this way.

The severe muscle loss is only the tip of the metabolic iceberg. Before substantial amounts of muscle evaporate, metabolism drops sharply as calories dip below maintenance levels. Only four days of caloric restriction suppresses all the major hormones responsible for burning body fat, maintaining energy levels and controlling hunger. The result: less energy is burned at rest and when active, less fat moves out of storage, more fat is stored in fat cells and hunger becomes unbearable. By day four you're already entrenched in a losing battle.

Not to be beaten, low-calorie advocates recommend a solution. Simply cut calories further. After all, this is low-calorie dieting. How low will you go? Before you realize, calories wither to such meager levels that decreasing them any further will jeopardize your health—as if you haven't already. And to be successful at maintaining your fat loss—you will not continue to lose, only maintain—your only choice remains severe calorie deprivation *for the rest of your life.*

Sounds like fun, doesn't it?

Low-Fat

Exciting news is quoted over and over in newspapers and magazines: Research shows low-fat dieters eat as much as they want and lose weight. New research? It must be true. Once again, you try low-fat dieting thinking of your failed attempts and bland food choices but motivated by the thought of eating as much as you want. You will succeed this time and you'll do everything to insure it, even if it means cutting fat calories to near zero. Dressing-less salads, fat-free pastries, pretzels, potatoes, pears and even popcorn—minus the butter, salt and taste—round out your menu. You discover pasta with fat-free spaghetti sauce, fat-free candy, fat-free cookies, fat-free chips and more. Even soft drinks are fat-free. It's been a week, time to check progress. You head back to your new friend, the bathroom scale. The numbers are in and...you gained three pounds. What the...? Your friend, the scale, wouldn't play such a cruel joke. What's going on? Science proves you can eat as much as you want while losing weight if fat calories are kept extremely low. Doesn't it?

✧✧✧

As a matter of fact, American consumers eat far less fat today than thirty years ago, but skyrocketing rates of obesity imply something mysterious about those all-you-can-eat studies. What do the studies really say? The technical classification of these smorgasbord-sounding studies is the Latin phrase *ad libitum.* Think of *ad libitum* as a way of saying the researchers and participants were too lazy to keep track of the calories. You can generate excitement by suggesting the subjects ate to their heart's content. On the other hand, you tell the real story by saying the subjects ate as little as they wanted—eating only low-fat foods proved difficult.

During low-fat diets, when participants and researchers actually recorded or controlled calorie intake, the only subjects experiencing weight loss were those cutting calories below maintenance levels. To sustain their weight loss, they suffer the same fate as those who start by cutting calories: eternal dieting. The apparent magic of all-you-can-eat, low-fat dieting comes from a clever spin on words or maybe a misunderstanding among reporters, not from the diet itself.

Familiarity with diet plans leaves few surprised by the truth: low-fat diets require calorie restriction to achieve weight loss. Cutting calories is simply an accepted part of the sacrifice. But choosing the low-fat method for weight loss means sacrificing more than just tasty treats and calories—you'll be sacrificing muscle. Of all the popular dietary schemes, none destroy more muscle than low-fat dieting. Over the first year, only 20% of a low-fat dieter's weight loss comes from body fat. Losing 50 lbs of weight means only 10 lbs of fat loss, with the majority of the balance from muscle. Eliminating dietary fat only magnifies the worst aspect of cutting calories— significantly less muscle loss occurs when cutting calories if dietary fat remains intact.

As if the negative impact of muscle loss on health isn't enough, there's more. Keeping levels of dietary fat below 10%—the recommendation of low-fat plans such as *The Pritikin Principle*—aims to reduce cholesterol levels, a task for which it performs well. Resolving this one feature of Syndrome X, however, is countered by increasing four, more deadly aspects of Syndrome X. Not only does a low-fat approach to weight loss jeopardize your health through muscle loss, but such severe dietary limits on fat accelerates the development of a syndrome known to shorten your life expectancy.

Ready to jump on the low-fat bandwagon?

Low-Carb

First no food, and then no fat and now it's no carbs. As you tell friends about your new diet you're warned about, no, almost threatened with a list of ailments: inability to think, bad breath, clogged arteries, obesity and cancer. Finally, your nutritionist strikes the deathblow—your body needs carbohydrates to live. Your head spins. How can all this be true when studies confirm the opposite? And you've never heard about anyone dying from not eating carbohydrates, but the idea is so new, nobody really knows much about these diets yet. Right?

❖❖❖

The low-carb diet—more properly, the ketogenic diet—is nothing new. The long and varied history began with a small publication written by…William Banting? That was 1863. You might have been thinking Dr Atkins, but his first book, *Dr Atkins' Diet Revolution*, wasn't published until over one hundred years later in 1972. And he was still preceded by three other versions of the low-carb diet, two of which made it to publication in the late '50s and early '60s. Even by then, another version emerged in the 1920s to fight childhood epilepsy and its use continues today. While not a pioneer, Dr Atkins did popularize the low-carb approach by allowing users to continually increase dietary carbohydrate levels. This simple change, as opposed to the strict lifelong limits associated with earlier versions, makes low-carb diets highly marketable—and very risky.

To avoid confusion, we need to identify a clear difference among these ketogenic diets and find a more useful phrase than ketogenic. Mainstream low-carb dieters restrict carbs to 50% or less of daily calories, hovering regularly near the top of the scale. Advocates don't normally explain it this way, but it appears to be the common thread. Scientific research, however, describes a more specific range from 8% to 50% of calories from carbs. This is about 40 to 250 grams per day. Anything less than 8%—specifically, 30 grams or less—falls under the heading *ultralow*-carb. Since these are both ketogenic diets, this may seem like splitting hairs, but the difference between the two is the difference between success and failure.

During an *ultralow*-carb diet, the body stops making some very special and bothersome enzymes. These enzymes convert carbohydrates into fat, which can then be stored as body fat. The ultralow-carb diet cuts off the one avenue available through which carbohydrates can become body fat, guaranteeing that an overdose of carbs has no possible way of heading to your stomach or thighs in the form of body fat. On the other hand, with their extra carb allowance, simple low-carb diets trigger the production of these carb-to-fat converting enzymes making it possible to store all those extra carbs you thought you were enjoying as fat.

As an example, Atkins begins as an ultralow-carb diet for two weeks, after which you slowly switch to the standard low-carb diet by adding fruits, vegetables and loads of sugar-alcohols (more about these later). Had Dr Atkins required

24

maintaining the ultralow portion for the next six months, you would enjoy ongoing and significant fat loss, even though the rate of fat loss would slow and eventually plateau. Instead, as carbs increase in the diet, so does body weight—as a matter of fact, by the end of the sixth month you've stopped losing body fat and started gaining. For us, for our goal of fat loss, this is the most important difference between these two ketogenic diets: ultralow-carb and simple low-carb.

The simple act of eating carbohydrates, even as little as 50 grams per day, prematurely stops fat loss and can accelerate body fat gain. Avoiding these problems takes 30 grams or less. Does adding more and more carbohydrates to your diet still seem like a blessing from Dr Atkins?

But we can't ignore the common fault: neither diet—low-carb or ultralow-carb—spikes insulin levels. This is incredibly important. The body produces the hormone insulin in response to a carb-rich meal; insulin then helps the body use carbohydrates for energy. Since both diets limit the intake of carbs, both diets limit the release of insulin. Low-carb enthusiasts flaunt this as an advantage, since elevated levels of insulin often mean little fat burning. An insulin spike, however, only temporarily stops fat burning, but the resulting hormonal afterglow accelerates body-fat burning for days.

Besides enhancing metabolism by itself, insulin also creastes a lasting glow by acting similar to a booster rocket. Booster rockets provide a short burst of extra force to propel some *thing*—airplane, satellite or space shuttle—before being ejected. In much the same way, a short and powerful burst of insulin boosts levels of several, to say the least, impressive fat burning hormones. Insulin levels plummet within two hours, but just as the space shuttle continues on without its booster rockets, the levels of these fat-burning hormones stay elevated for nearly four days. Also like the space shuttle, which would never get off the ground without the booster rockets, these crucial hormones will *never* accelerate fat burning without an insulin spike.

Insulin and Hormone Spikes

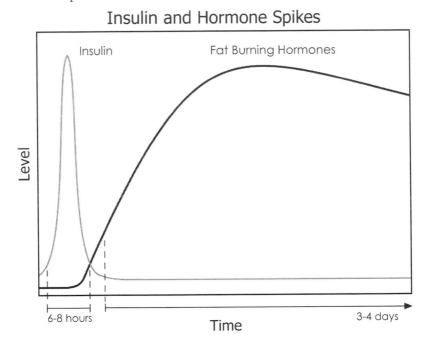

Of the several hormones affected by insulin spikes, leptin may be the most important. Leptin telegraphs information about body fat reserves and calorie intake throughout the body, acting like a fatness and nutrient thermostat. Normally, when fat cells are full and our bodies get enough food, leptin levels are high; as a result, we can lose body fat. But if fat cells empty or calories fall too low, leptin levels also fall. In addition, research shows that stripping carbs from the diet causes leptin levels to plunge, no matter how much fat and protein you eat. Actually, leptin levels mimic the lows found in starvation when carbs are lacking. And low leptin levels signal fat cells to stay full and store as much incoming fat as possible—in other words: kiss your fat loss good bye. This may explain why several years of maintaining low insulin levels causes unavoidable fat gain—even for those eating only carbs causing small amounts of insulin release. Fat loss and even weight maintenance are nearly hopeless without periodic insulin spikes. Unfortunately, as neither the ultralow-carb nor low-carb diet offers any hope of spiking insulin levels, there appears no way to overcome this fatal problem while clinging to the requirements of these diets.

Dr Atkins claims a low-carb diet creates a metabolic advantage. What do you think?

Low Glycemic Index

A new wave hits the diet industry and you soon find yourself swimming in conversations laced with phrases from, apparently, another language. You search for meaning in the expressions *low-glycemic index carbohydrate* and *high-glycemic index carbohydrate*. Relief comes when you learn simply that some carbs are good and some bad. But there are also friendly carbs, which sound good as well. When you search through the different food lists you make a startling discovery: some good carbs aren't friendly, some bad carbs are. You learn more and the confusion only mounts. Can the glycemic index do anything other than complicate your life?

✧✧✧

As acceptance fades among medical professionals, the glycemic index (GI) moves to the field of weight loss for a second chance at life. Before diving into a technical discussion about what glycemic index means, how it's used, the difference between high- and low-GI, friendly, or good and bad carbs, the scientific research sums up the fat loss and even health claims with a single word: nonsense.

Rather than restricting carbohydrates altogether, reliance on glycemic index for menu choice approaches the same goal as low-carb diets: insulin control. Like low-carb diets, low-GI diets focus on limiting insulin release because insulin can stop the body from burning fat. The truth: *Simply eating carbohydrates, alone or in combination with other nutrients, prevents your body from burning fat regardless of how much or how little insulin levels rise.*

Glycemic index diets recommend eating low-GI carbs, which create the smallest rise in blood sugar levels and, normally, the lowest rise in insulin. Unfortunately, low-GI carbs also stop you from burning fat for the longest periods because low-GI carbs cause the longest periods of elevated blood sugar and insulin levels. And some of the lowest GI carbs are undeniably the most fattening of all. Yes, low-glycemic carbs are the supposed 'good' ones—good for what? Nobody knows as researchers continually fail to find a connection between low-GI diets and weight loss, or a connection between high-GI diets and weight gain.

Despite the absence of a connection between low-GI diets and weight loss, a link to weight gain—specifically, fat gain—does exist. Similar to low-carb diets, a low-GI diet fails to spike insulin levels, causing metabolism to slow over the years and body fat storage to increase. With low-carb diets, less than a year passes before this slow, consistent weight gain settles in, but low-GI diets may take several years before landing you in this situation. Although the time frames differ, the result is identical: a slow, steady gain of a few pounds of body-fat per year. According to research, you can do little to stop the process while meticulously following the strict low-GI guidelines as recommended by The Zone, Sugar Busters!®, Fat Flush® and even South Beach.

Do you still believe South Beach will get you into a Speedo® swimsuit as the diet implies?

Mini-Meals

Wow! You finally learned the secret: eat six meals per day and lose weight. The idea makes perfect sense: going too long between meals scares the body into storing excess body fat. But eating every three hours relaxes the body and the weight melts away. It's so simple. You plan for the next day with plenty of time for preparing easy-travel meals. Before you realize, work's piled up and you scurry every morning to put your meals together. This week's even worse and you settle for the cafeteria, nutrition bars, vending machines and, heaven forbid, fast food restaurants. Eating went from enjoyable to irritating, but the results are worth it, right? That cover-model body is just around the corner. You've been watching your weight for weeks now and it's down two pounds one week, up one the next, maybe the same the week after that, then down, then...well, it's just not changing much at all. You're not losing weight, eating is a full time job and missing one meal sends hunger pains off the chart. How did you get into this mess?

✧✧✧

Trying to discover the perfect number of daily meals for health and weight loss has been going on since the 1950s and the vast majority of studies—32 of the 36—reveal this conclusive result regarding weight loss: the ideal number of meals per day is...whatever you feel like. Whether you eat one, two, three, all the way up to six or more meals per day you'll lose exactly the same amount of body fat, keep exactly the same amount of muscle and, therefore, end up with identical weight loss but *only* by restricting calories. If daily calories are kept low and equal, say 1200, identical fat loss occurs with one 1200-calorie meal per day, or three 400-calorie meals per day, or even six 200-calorie meals per day. Regardless of the number of meals, the previously discussed problems of calorie restriction are unavoidable—muscle loss, falling metabolism, and fat cell buildup.

The studies prove a few more interesting things. First, consuming several smaller meals throughout the day actually lowers metabolism over time: even without calorie restriction, the ill effects of a low-calorie diet materialize from spreading meals thin. Secondly, a powerful hunger-stimulating hormone called ghrelin establishes a strict eating schedule. Forcing yourself to stick with a rigid and frequent eating schedule eventually triggers rising ghrelin levels prior to each mealtime, causing extreme hunger pangs. Besides ravenous cravings, missing a regularly scheduled meal results in sluggishness and irritation. Finally, having to eat more than three times per day brought complaints from nearly every study subject about the difficulty of scheduling so many meals—even when meals were prepared for them.

Just what you've always wanted in a weight loss plan: slower metabolism; increased hunger; difficult scheduling; all with no benefits. Ready to start eating every three hours?

Exercise for Weight Loss

Exercise sounded foolproof. With all those svelte, reedy runners and lean, buff bicyclists it must work. Everyday you pull yourself from the warmth of the bed to begin those chilled morning runs. You even welcome free afternoons with a little burned rubber from the new bicycle. The weather sometimes forces you to the treadmill or stationary bike, but you don't mind—the whirring motors lull you into your zone. Six months of unwavering dedication and you're shocked by the results: you've lost four pounds. Four pounds? You fume after remembering all those wasted hours running and cycling to lose less than one pound a month. How can you spend so much time, expend so much energy and lose so little weight?

✧✧✧

Being nearly as old a recommendation as low-fat, exercise often replaces diet as a way to lose weight. Who better to follow than those already there? Professional distance runners and cyclists, along with other elite endurance athletes, maintain a small, toned figure throughout their careers, which many began as children. And this is the key: they've always been thin, slim and trim. Never in their lives did they need to lose body fat. When using exercise, any type of exercise for weight loss—including running, cycling, weight lifting, walking, bouncing—the average person is lucky to lose one pound a month. For the first six months, it's normally less. Don't expect those few pounds to be fat, either. After a large group

31

attempted exercise for fat loss, the results led researchers to advise waiting at least *nine full months* before hoping to see any fat loss resulting from exercise—nine full months of zero fat loss.

As time goes on, the research only becomes more convincing. Comparing those who start diet and exercise with those who only diet reveals both groups lose identical amounts of weight—exercise contributed nothing to the loss. Taking it a step further, comparing those who begin exercise without a diet plan with those who just sit around all day still shows identical weight loss, which is zilch in this case—again, exercise contributed nothing. Even those trying to maintain their newly achieved figures failed when using exercise without diet—once again, nothing. And unlike those trying to convince you with one or two studies that exercise will help you lose body fat, over two-dozen studies show exercise doesn't help fat loss sooner than six months into your routine. Although many compelling reasons to exercise exist, short-term fat loss is not one of them.

Still planning on running to help get you into that swimsuit by spring?

A Good Start

We Have a Winner

You've been reading this book in the hopes of learning how to rid your body of those annoying fat deposits and, so far, the entire discussion has detailed what's wrong with everything else. By now, I hope you're convinced to at least try a different approach. But the current options seem useless for fat loss, so what's left?

Returning to the primary goal, which is weight loss while sparing muscle, there's only one option to reconsider—the ultralow-carb option. In a diet containing high levels of carbohydrates, if carb supplies ever fade too quickly—such as eating too little or during exercise—muscle is converted into sugar for energy. Muscles continue wasting away until the body receives a fresh supply of carbohydrates or no longer needs any. While not always perfect, low-carb diets stop muscles from being destroyed for energy.

When low-carb plans keep carbohydrates low enough and dietary fat high enough, the resulting change in metabolism makes the body more comfortable burning fat for energy as opposed to muscle. Carbohydrate levels must be kept consistently minimal because the body always prefers carbs, and once these run out on a carb-rich diet, muscle becomes the next source of energy. As a carb-restricted diet wears on, muscle remains safest from destruction when dietary carbohydrates are lowest, making the ultralow-carb diet an excellent starting point for a fat loss plan.

Besides sparing muscle, the ultralow-carb diet provides several other advantages. Not only does the ultralow-carb diet avoid some of the physical stress associated with dieting—meaning lower cortisol levels—there is little insulin around to initiate the growth of new fat cells. The very nature of the ultralow-carb diet keeps both insulin and cortisol levels extremely low, making it immune to the most disastrous side effect of traditional diets.

The ultralow-carb diet also controls hunger more readily than other types of diets. Contrary to popular belief, insulin is not the most potent hunger-stimulating hormone. Actually, insulin's role in stimulating hunger is poorly understood. The current theory involving insulin (as explained in South Beach, Atkins and other soures) lacks conclusive evidence. A newly discovered hormone, ghrelin, stimulates hunger more than any other. When ghrelin levels are high, hunger rises and when levels fall, so do the cravings. Carbohydrates cause a crash in ghrelin levels immediately after a meal, delivering a feeling of satisfaction, but a carb-based diet also causes ghrelin to spike between meals making hunger extremely powerful. The ultralow-carb diet avoids this problem by keeping ghrelin levels under control—levels are never too high and most often low.

The other major problem when dieting is the plunge in metabolic rate, which is also partially avoided with the ultralow-carb diet. Your basal metabolic rate—the rate at which your body burns energy when resting—slowly falls on an ultralow-carb diet instead of plummeting within the first week, as occurs with typical diets. Regrettably, problems with leptin levels falling still persist and metabolism will drop. Of paramount importance is finding some way to avoid these two problems or those fat cells will never empty. And if they do, a plateau will quickly develop.

The real trick is finding some way to preserve or even increase metabolism and levels of fat burning hormones like leptin. Resolving this problem not only guarantees ongoing fat loss, but also makes a rebound unlikely.

A Painful Epiphany

Having just completed my Master's work in Physics, I decided to try my first bodybuilding contest. This wasn't my first attempt at getting into contest shape. Several times before, diet and exercise were combined in the hopes of seeing my abdominal muscles. All prior attempts ended in failure—no diet had ever worked as advertised. I began to believe my body would always be against me. So, this was my last ditch effort.

At the time, the only diet with any promise of dropping my body fat levels to minimum was the ultralow-carb diet. Other amateur bodybuilders chose a low-fat, ultralow-carb diet, but my research showed that higher levels of fat are important. Research at the medical library also supported the promise of saving as much muscle as possible during the weight loss. I'd tried it once before without success. This time I convinced myself it would work. I ate nothing but eggs, ground beef, chicken, cheeses, and oils.

Sticking to the diet became difficult after the first week, but I continued for five more. Then, late one night, I had a run in with a couple of dozen donuts. I still remember the smell of those warm, freshly made Krispy Kremes® as I slipped into a mindless feeding frenzy. Within minutes, 20 donuts disappeared. Shortly after emerging from the zombie-like state, I found myself curled in the fetal position. Prior to falling asleep—or maybe passing out—I moaned from the stomachache.

The next morning I collected myself and recommitted to preparing for the bodybuilding competition. I noticed a little bloating, otherwise the damage looked minor. I returned to my regimen of meats, cheeses and oils. By the next day there were no signs of the donut disaster. On the third morning a rush of excitement hit. The first ever appearance of my abs made it clear, I was ahead of schedule—farther than I'd ever dreamed. I repeated a less painful variation of the donut disaster once a week to achieve the chiseled physique needed to win the contest. The Carb Nite Solution was born.

Over the next couple of years, I invested the majority of my time researching why this worked. In the process, the diet has been highly refined—nearly perfected. And it turned out to be simpler than ever imagined and held further surprises.

Introducing The Carb Nite™ Solution

The Carb Nite™ Solution

Believe it or not, it takes only one small modification to the ultralow-carb diet to make it nearly the perfect fat stripping diet: a Carb Nite. The Carb Nite Solution is the magic pill for creating the key for rapid fat loss. Here's the entire dietary plan from start to finish.

Reorientation:
For the first nine days keep carbohydrates to 30 grams or less per day—equivalent to two slices of white bread; only fiber does not count as a carbohydrate in this total. Eat enough food to keep hunger under control without worrying about counting calories.

Carb Nite:
Day ten starts off like the previous nine days but starting at around dinner time (sometime between 4 and 6 pm) you must eat a sizable amount of carbs: spaghetti, apricots, pie, potato-chips, bread, bananas, bagels, donuts, ice-cream, cookies, cheesecake and almost anything else you've been craving. You should eat carbs for the rest of the evening—this includes all the way until bedtime and maybe even a midnight snack.

Day after your first Carb Nite:
Go back to 30 grams or less of carbohydrates per day—the same as your first nine days.

Long Haul:
For up to six months you continue this cycle of having a Carb Nite at least once per week, but you must keep them at least four full days apart. For instance, if you have a Carb Nite on Friday, you cannot have your next Carb Nite any sooner than Wednesday.

The Rules

At the base of this program clearly lies the ultralow-carb diet. Any diet grappling with fat loss should be based on the ultralow-carb diet—not low-calorie, not low-fat and not simply low-carb. This is important: the only compelling results confirming fat loss while preserving muscle come from limiting carbohydrate intake to 30 grams or less per day—some people even gain a little muscle. Other diets can't boast this kind of scientific support and therefore conflict with our primary goal of fat loss, rather than simple weight loss.

Up to this point, the amount of dietary fat in the ultralow-carb scheme has remained unspecified. You need to understand: cutting carbs to near zero levels is not our only concern. The amount of dietary fat is also crucial. Eating low-carb *and* low-fat—in other words, high protein—has no advantages, but possesses the same drawbacks as a low-fat, low-calorie diet, with one difference. Eating high levels of protein without enough fat or carbohydrates actually accelerates the rate of muscle loss. To avoid muscle loss, ultralow-carb plans require relatively high levels of dietary fat for full advantage. Tools for insuring proper amounts of fat in comparison with protein, accompanied by an explanation are in the Food Lists section.

> ➢ Rule 1: Eat plenty of fat

An ultralow-carb diet, unfortunately, requires some sort of adjustment period at the start. To insure maximum benefits, many changes need to take place—changes that only take place one at a time. Being strict those first few days empties carbohydrate stores, at which point the brain begins gearing up to use an alternative fuel instead of the normal carbohydrates.

C   Also during this time, the enzymes for turning carbs into fat are no longer produced and existing levels dwindle. On average, the entire Reorientation process runs about seven days, but can last up to ten. So, erring on the side of caution and enduring nine days with minimal carbs guarantees maximum boost from the first Carb Nite.

Day 10—a day of reckoning for most people. It's the first Carb Nite experience, ever, and it's bound to include a few surprises, inspire a little excitement, and instill a subtle anxiety. But for the most part, it's fun and, more importantly, critical to your success. Although the ultralow-carb diet fends off the drop in metabolism better than most diets, it still suffers a slow fall along with an abrupt drop in fat burning hormones.

D   Remarkably, one 6-8 hour Carb Nite completely reverses the trend by spiking metabolism and raising levels of all the major fat burning hormones, including leptin. Carb Nite even ignites excess fat burning. After the weeklong absence of carbs, these effects shadow soaring insulin levels, but unlike insulin levels, which fall within a few hours, metabolism and levels of all the fat burning hormones stay elevated for the next *four days*. After the fourth day everything tends to fall again, making Carb Nite a vital weekly ritual while on The Carb Nite Solution.

Don't think that eating a piece of bread once a week will produce these fat-stripping hormonal and metabolic changes. Carb Nite only works as a metabolism booster by eating a substantial amount of carbs over the course of an evening.

E   We're talking mashed potatoes, pasta, custard, cookies, apricots, angel food, eggnog, éclairs, bagels and bread. And don't forget a source of protein from chicken, beef, pork, eggs, milk, fish or some other, preferably, lean source. This amounts to little more than a typical meal complete with dessert. Both carbs and protein are important for the positive mental effects as for the fat-burning and muscle-sparing boost. Moreover, feel free to splurge on the carbs without guilt. Remember, your body will no longer be capable of turning carbs into body fat for the evening. It's exceedingly difficult to store body fat on Carb Nite, so live it up.

Keep in mind it's Carb Nite, not Carb Meal. Stimulating the metabolic changes responsible for ongoing fat loss requires more than a single meal—even an extremely large one. Six to eight hours of eating carbohydrates creates the hormonal afterglow we're seeking, but a single carb meal only elevates metabolism for the evening, an effect incapable of accelerating fat loss. Rather than a single meal, try an early supper and a late dinner together with a before-bed snack. Or maybe you'd rather snack before a big meal while delaying the pumpkin pie à la mode for later in the night. You don't need to eat extremely large amounts of food per sitting—although you can if you choose—simple snacking throughout the evening often achieves the goal. Enjoy the entire, possibly gluttonous, night.

> Rule 2: Enjoy a *full* Carb Nite.

Now that you're done with Carb Nite, it's back to 30 grams of carbs a day for the next six or so days. Choosing the day of your next Carb Nite now depends on convenience as much as science. There are only two more rules. Rule three: Never skip Carb Nite. Carb Nite keeps the body in a constant state of accelerated body-fat burning. Skipping a Carb Nite amounts to little more than slowing fat loss and pointless self-torture. The complexity of the human body makes predicting a minimum rate of fat loss impossible. On this, or any plan, expect some weeks to bring greater fat loss than others, especially if relying on a bathroom scale to track progress. The Carb Nite Solution is the most advanced fat loss diet, but periodically a week may pass where the numbers on the scale don't change—especially when reaching extremely low levels of body fat. But don't skip Carb Nite under the assumption of accelerating fat loss. Missing a weekly Carb Nite creates an immediate plateau. No matter the goal, avoiding Carb Nite only puts it farther out of reach. Carb Nite is a once-per-week *obligation*.

> ➢ Rule 3: Never skip Carb Nite.

Finally, the fourth rule: Never have Carb Nite sooner than the fifth night after your last Carb Nite. Since hormone levels begin slipping by this time, it might seem tempting to give them a kick, but the body needs at least four full days to shed any stored carbs from the last Carb Nite and levels of the carb-to-fat converting enzymes need just as long to fade. So, enjoying carbs again before the fifth night could add body fat while crippling the hormonal spike. Carb Nite is a once-per-week *proposition*.

> ➢ Rule 4: Never have Carb Nite sooner than the fifth night after your last one.

Carb Nite, the literal guilt-free, carbohydrate indulgence, solves the problem of falling metabolism and hormones, clearly showing why Carb Nite is the key to the success of this plan. Carb Nite, however, gives so much more. All previous diets fail to prevent a rebound—diet forever or gain all the weight back, and then some. The Carb Nite Solution differs greatly by keeping the body constantly bewildered. The choice of an ultralow-carb diet first confuses the body into perceiving starvation while getting plenty of food. Secondly, after every Carb Nite, fat cells become extremely disoriented: the low levels of insulin together with skyrocketed levels of leptin instruct fat cells to empty out while already being empty. With typical diets, this combination of events rarely, if ever, happens and the hormonal-mixed signals may lead the body to do something drastic: *kill fat cells.* This is the first diet program naturally creating a hormonal environment proven to kill fat cells in animals. Unlike other diet plans that create more fat cells—specifically low-calorie and low-fat diets—The Carb Nite Solution may destroy them, closing the door on the chance of a rebound. You've been battling long enough, isn't it time to finally win the war?

Be aware: the road to victory has pit stops. With all good things come limits and The Carb Nite Solution is no exception. Because of the power carried by these hormonal changes, the body may eventually adapt and become temporarily resistant to some of the more remarkable effects. In addition, few studies on the ultralow-carb diet span periods greater than six months, and although promising, there are still too few to make accurate, scientific recommendations on extended use. For these two reasons, The Carb Nite Solution is to be cycled— up to six months on with at least a month off before restarting. You'll whittle away body-fat until reaching your ultimate goal, no matter how slim and trim you desire to become, each time becoming slimmer, happier and healthier than before.

To Count, or Not to Count; That Is the Question

Hopefully, you noticed the advice to abstain from counting calories—many people welcome the suggestion. The age-old practice of counting calories seems to be a veritable rite of passage for those serious about weight loss. But we're not here to simply lose weight; we're here to strip fat, and like many other accepted norms, we're casting aside the ritual of calorie counting. Ignoring the establishment is not done lightly: the idea behind counting calories actually violates the laws of physics.

Keeping an accurate account of daily calories makes sense only if the body gets the same amount of energy from 100 calories of carbohydrates as 100 calories of fat as 100 calories of protein. But it doesn't. Because food requires energy to process, some of the ingested calories get wasted. Eating 100 calories of fat leaves your body with only 97 calories by the time it's finished processing; 100 calories of carbs leaves the body with 93 calories to use; 100 calories of protein gives the body only 70 calories. For perspective, two meals, one high in carbs and the other high in protein, could both contain 340 calories according to labels. As far as the body is concerned, the high-carb meal delivers 316 calories, but the high-protein meal only makes 238 calories available.

Even if you want to go through the calculations, making all the necessary adjustments for each nutrient, your arithmetic won't always add up. Not only do different nutrients provide differing calories from those listed on labels, sometimes the same nutrient can provide differing calorie counts. While in many situations fat only supplies 9 calories per gram, there are times when fat supplies up to 11 calories per gram. Just like a car achieving 18 miles per gallon for in-town driving and 26 miles per gallon for interstate driving, the body runs more efficiently at times and gets more distance out of food. Unfortunately, there's no practical way of knowing exactly when your body is being more efficient.

The human body is just too adaptive, too efficient and too unpredictable to count calorie usage accurately. It's extremely naïve to believe that counting numbers on the back of a cereal box is enough to predict how one of the most complex machines in the world is going to respond—although many nutrition and health experts still insist. The total energy intake—normally measured as calories—is important, but no convenient and reliable way of measuring exists. Your best bet is to follow the guidelines set forth in this book while making certain to control hunger. It's the best *anyone* can do.

A Little Word About Food

You are what you eat—literally. Everything about the health and performance of your body, right down to individual cells, depends on what you eat. I assume some familiarity with the subject of food, such as the difference between carbs, protein and fat. Understanding the best food choices for this diet requires a little extra information, but not much. This section is by no means exhaustive on the subject of food, nor is that the intent. Without weighing you down—or boring you—with an over-abundance of information, this section explains the necessities for success on The Carb Nite Solution and hopefully demystifies a few terms floating around in the media and on nutrition labels.

Fat

From years of relentless vilification, dietary fat suffers a terrible stigma. Though some of us know better, we still cringe at the thought of buttered bread, filet mignon, bacon and sometimes, even nuts. We shouldn't. Fat is an important part of the diet. It's the type of dietary fat we need to concern ourselves with.

Recent diets present fat as an alternative to carbohydrates for fueling the body. Several parallels exist between the ways the body uses carbs and fat, but the differences are more interesting. Fats have between twice to three times the amount of energy per gram. Where carbs are available for energy almost immediately after a meal, fat takes between two and six hours. But most importantly, the body needs dietary fat to survive, while carbs remain optional. Lacking the ability to create certain fats, your body relies completely on diet to supply them, making fat an essential nutrient.

Saturated

Saturated fat is found mostly in animal products like butter, meat and cheese and is typically solid at room temperature. Normally considered extremely harmful, according to research this mainly holds true if you're eating large amounts of saturated fat in a diet containing large amounts of carbohydrates. When you strip carbs from the diet there seem to be few health consequences from eating saturated fat—at least, short-term consequences. And at least one type of saturated fat positively affects health, regardless of diet. For you chocolate aficionados: over a third of the saturated fat in cocoa butter is the healthy kind.

As for any type of diet, getting your fats from primarily saturated sources is a bad idea. So whether eating carbs or not, eat saturated fat in moderation to avoid developing a bad habit. Only worry about avoiding saturated fats during the first meal of your Carb Nites—skipping out on a piece of cheesecake for dessert later in the evening is a tad extreme. Remember: live a little.

Monounsaturated

Monounsaturated fat is the main fat in olive, canola, almond and several other plant oils. As with all oils, it's liquid at room temperature. Because monounsaturated fat remains stable at high temperatures, it's excellent for frying and other types of cooking.

Normally praised for the ability to reverse several metabolic problems and help weight loss efforts, monounsaturated fat hides a dark secret: a friendship with fat cells. No other type of fat fills fat cells more easily. And once inside, monounsaturated fat doesn't come back out easily. Overeating monounsaturated fat, especially with carbs, can refill empty fat cells in a flash, rapidly accelerating body-fat gain. The many health benefits of monounsaturated fat come when eating a moderate to low calorie, often, high-fiber diet. If taking guidance from the included Meal Plans, which helps to avoid overeating, then choose monounsaturated fat over saturated when possible: it is, in general, healthier. Too much olive oil on Carb Nite creates the most common hazard from monounsaturated fat.

Polyunsaturated

By far, the healthiest fats are polyunsaturated. They can also be found in plant oils like almond, flax and canola and, in addition, several rich animal sources like cold-water fish, grass-fed or grazing livestock, wild game and even eggs. Because they break down into other types of fat when heated, don't use oils, such as flax, for high-temperature cooking like broiling or frying.

The polyunsaturated fats divide into omega-3's and omega-6's, both of which are essential in the diet—the body manufactures saturated and monounsaturated fats, but cannot manufacture omega-3's or 6's. Not only does your health depend on eating enough polyunsaturated fat, but also on a balance of the two types. Currently, you probably consume about 10 to 25 times as much omega-6 fat as omega-3 while the optimum ratio is thought to lie somewhere around three to one. You may be getting nearly nine times the amount of needed omega-6's.

My recommendation to you is this: no matter what your dietary plan, supplement with as much omega-3 fat as possible. Your normal diet provides more than enough omega-6's and supplementation together with careful food selection is, unfortunately, the only real chance of correcting the imbalance. The appendix contains a list of common oils and the amount of omega-3's in comparison with omega-6's. The diet plans take this into account and help guide your food choices to get the largest health benefit from The Carb Nite Solution—this includes attempting to balance the polyunsaturated fats.

Trans-Fats

Mysterious sounding trans-fats carry with them a fair amount of confusion because, although studied for decades, the general public has only been exposed to the term recently. Trans-fats share many of the health-destroying effects of saturated fat and may even be worse. But not all trans-fats are bad, as many naturally occurring trans-fats possess health benefits. Hiding behind the names CLA and CLnA, these can be found in beef, safflower oil and some exotic seeds and nuts.

Artificial trans-fats, which make up about 3% of the American diet, pose the greatest health risk. Margarines and bakery type foods—like cakes, cookies and pies—make about 75% of all dietary sources of artificial trans-fats.

The greatest health threat comes from long-term, high dietary levels of trans-fats, which your body tends to store in such circumstances. Even with large stores, you can easily tame the threat. The body quickly releases trans-fats from fat cells and burns it for energy, so eliminating the main sources from your diet swiftly drains the unwanted stockpile. Avoiding trans-fats on The Carb Nite Solution is easy since the majority of products contain large amounts of carbohydrates. Exercise the most restraint on Carb Nites.

Protein

Like fat, protein is an essential nutrient. Amino acids are the building blocks of proteins forming long chains that make up enzymes, hormones, muscle and connective tissue in the body. If amino acids don't occur in the correct amounts in a protein, the body can't use it for any of the critical applications above, so proteins divide into two groups: complete and incomplete. Choosing your protein sources wisely gets into a long and complex discussion about quality ratings, amino acid profiles, food balancing and all sorts of other, dry subjects. The list below provides just enough information to make a huge difference in your diet with a minimum of detail.

Animal Proteins

As you might guess, these are proteins derived from animal products like meat, fish, eggs and dairy products. Animal proteins are by far your best protein choice and are complete. Your main source of protein should be from animal sources on The Carb Nite Solution.

Plant Proteins

Almost all plant proteins are incomplete. Without great care, several unpleasant deficiencies occur when trying to get your protein needs from only plant sources. The one common, complete protein from a plant source, soy, contains several additional chemicals that slow fat burning and hinder the body's ability to process protein, so it's an extremely poor choice on a diet designed specifically for fat loss while preserving muscle. Consequently, plant proteins are always a poor primary source of dietary protein—especially soy protein.

Whey Protein

Besides Little Miss Muffet eating her curds and whey, you may have never heard about whey protein. Whey protein comes from milk, but gets destroyed during pasteurization, leaving little available in the average diet. Coming from milk, it's obviously an animal protein, but because of its special properties and absence in the diet, whey protein deserves a spotlight.

There's no hope of increasing dietary whey protein other than with supplementation, but whey protein benefits the body in such a variety of ways you should to go to the trouble. Without getting into the several reasons for including whey protein in any type of diet, here's why you absolutely want a daily serving while on The Carb Nite Solution: whey protein preserves and helps build muscle, particularly during periods of weight loss—one of our primary goals.

Additionally, you'll find very few sources of antioxidants when developing new dietary habits after shedding carbs. Supplements like multivitamins help, but whey protein pushes the envelope on anti-oxidant protection. Instead of a few random molecules floating around, how would you feel about giving every cell in your body the most advanced and potent antioxidant weaponry? Actually, your cells already have the antioxidant machinery but need the correct ammunition, which whey protein provides in abundance. With a single, daily serving of whey protein every cell in your body is armed to the teeth against oxidative damage.

Could a more tailor made food for The Carb Nite Solution possibly exist? Doubtful, but remember to choose your supplements wisely. Search for pure whey protein isolate—as opposed to concentrate—in *powder* form, as it contains no carbohydrates and escapes pasteurization.

Carbohydrates

Saving the discussion on carbs for last is an easy decision. For starters, carbs are the only nutrient we can live without. Health experts, nutritionists and even some doctors often counter with, "The brain can only use carbohydrates for energy." Even if this were true, the body produces all the carbohydrates it can possibly need from protein—problem solved. But it's not true. Granted, up until 1967 it was a

51

commonly held belief. In 1967, however, the brain was discovered to use an alternative source of fuel called ketones, which the body manufactures from fat. Considering the stubbornness of the common misconception that the brain needs carbs to survive, many doctors, nutritionists, athletic trainers and celebrities posing as fitness experts would do well to sit down and learn about the wonderful advances in scientific knowledge since the late '60s.

The second reason for placing carbs last in the food discussion is the lingering confusion and mystery in classifying carbs properly for health. Scientists seek simplicity when dreaming up new theories; this may explain why the attempts at classifying carbs all have exactly two categories. Choices thus far have been: simple or complex, low-glycemic or high-glycemic, good or bad, and, standing as a monument to minimalism, Dr Phil's high-cost-low-yield or low-cost-high-yield. Chemists like the terms simple and complex, and diabetics use the term glycemic, but everyone else needs a different scheme. If, perchance, the number of categories can be raised to three, a perfectly suited classification exists that takes several factors into account at once: ability to stop fat burning, ability to trigger the production and storage of fat, ability to produce positive hormonal changes, ability to increase metabolism and ability to satiate. The following categories do not give the green light to overeating any one group. Overeating carbs or fat will make you fat—there is no food classification in the world to avoid this problem.

Fiber

The first carbohydrate category is fiber. Beside chemical similarities, fiber and other carbohydrates have little else in common—there are even dietary fibers that aren't carbohydrates. And, unlike other carbs, fiber basically does nothing in the body—no hormonal changes, no changes in metabolism, and provides no energy—until reaching the colon. Once there, beneficial bacteria ferment fiber, releasing fat in the process. You did read correctly: the body eventually metabolizes fiber as fat, healthy fat. Fiber slows digestion and promotes regular bowel movements and is implicated in the prevention of several types of cancer. For all these reasons include carbs from this group—pure fiber—into all days of The Carb Nite Solution. Fiber is excluded from the daily carb count because the body, with a little bacterial assistance, turns fiber into fat. You can and should eat as much fiber as it takes to keep you regular, both on and off this diet.

Although fiber is a low-GI carb, the advantages of a diet high in fiber are wrongly applied to diets high in any type of low-GI food. Fiber is extremely low on the GI spectrum—zero, actually—and the more you eat, the thinner you are. From here, cavalier assumptions about *all* low-GI carbs quickly swept the marketplace. *Fiber is the only carbohydrate, low-GI or otherwise, conclusively associated with reduced body-fat when eaten throughout life.*

Bulk Carbohydrate Sweeteners

The food manufacturing and diet industry can be thanked for discovering this category and determining which carbohydrates to include. As the name implies, these carbohydrates are used in large quantities to sweeten everything from soft drinks to cakes and even chewing gum. The Bulk Carbohydrate Sweeteners are fructose, high-fructose corn syrup, glycerin and sugar alcohols and cause reactions not normally associated with eating carbs. Like fiber, Bulk Carbohydrate Sweeteners are also extremely low-glycemic, but unlike fiber Bulk Carbohydrate Sweeteners:

- Can lower insulin levels
- Stop fat burning
- Increase fat production
- Surge production of the carb-to-fat converting enzymes
- Lower leptin levels
- Fail to lower ghrelin levels
- Slow metabolism
- Cause diabetes.

Consequently, the bulk sweeteners make you sluggish, create the perfect environment for accelerating fat gain, paralyze the ability to burn body fat and are completely incapable of satisfying hunger. Avoid this group of carbs at all times—they will only make you fat. Items with high concentrations are easily identified: soft drinks, fruit juice, "junk food" and nearly all meal replacement bars, especially those with a Net Carb, Impact Carb or Effective Carb label.

Classical Carbs

Think of Classical Carbs as everything leftover after excluding fiber and bulk carbohydrate sweeteners. Traditional labels are difficult to use because the group includes both simple and complex carbohydrates, as well as both low- and high-glycemic carbs and there are most likely a few low-cost-high-yield carbs sprinkled throughout.

Classical Carbs produce the effects most often thought of as carb-like: elevated insulin and blood sugar levels, and boosted energy. Current dieting philosophy labels these carbs as bad and blames everything from obesity to diabetes on eating these classics. In their attempts to disgrace Classical Carbs, current experts ignore the most powerful effects: increasing metabolism, burning fat (once insulin levels fall), satisfying hunger and raising leptin levels. Insulin spikes—which everyone thinks dreadful—accelerate metabolism, initiate the emptying of fat cells and prevent long-term weight gain. Does this sound wicked to you? These spikes ultimately tell fat cells to empty out and reveal the figure you've been dieting to see. And the Bulk Carbohydrate Sweeteners have been proven to accelerate diabetes, not the Classical Carbs. By focusing solely on the very short-term effects of insulin, the current popular carb classification demonizes the wrong carbs. Classical Carbs will account for the majority of your food on Carb Nite and are easy to find, as you're already familiar with these truly "good" carbs: bread, bananas, pasta, potatoes, granola, grenadine, biscuits, bagels, scones, skewers, and corn—yellow and white, kernel and creamed, and even popped. This, by the way, is a tiny list of your options.

Nutrition Labels

The ability to read nutrition labels, to recognize and filter out worthwhile information, is invaluable on this or any diet plan. The labels look simple, but despite the best efforts of the United States Food and Drug Administration to make a standardized, easy to understand label, deciphering one is not easy.

Basic Layout

Let's take a look at a typical label. It's broken up into three primary areas, followed by the list of ingredients. The top most area gives the serving size and the amount of calories present in one serving. The middle section breaks the item down into the amount present, in grams, of the three basic nutrients: fat, carbohydrates and protein. The bottom section gives extra, optional information, which is normally helpful in pointing out any additional health-promoting properties. Or, at least, those things marketers want you to believe healthy or special. You'll notice the last two sections contain percentages on the far right-hand side.

Anatomy of a Nutrition Label

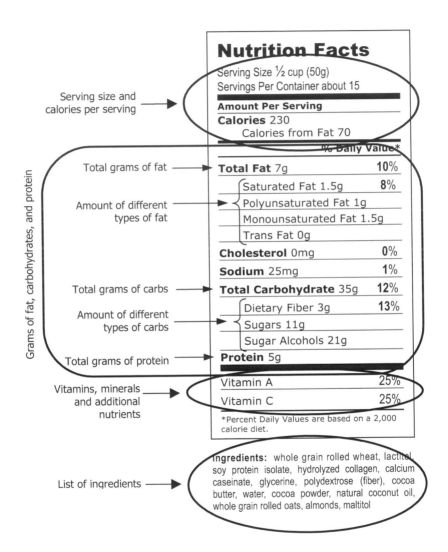

The middle section deserves careful attention because it's the heart of the nutritional information. The section displays all the important information about the food. Not only are grams of fat listed, but the type of fat as well. Typically, only the amount of saturated fat is listed; if you're lucky, mono-unsaturated fat and polyunsaturated fats will also be listed. You may find the monounsaturated fat listed as omega-9 along with polyunsaturated fats broken down into the amount of omega-3's and omega-6's, which is the best you can hope for in the fat section of a nutrition label. Trans-fats, too, will probably make an appearance under the fat section once labeling requirements are updated. Finding a label with all this information about fat content is a stroke of luck.

The carbohydrate section also contains an apparent cornucopia of information. Like fats, the total number of grams is listed with a break down of the types of carbs underneath. You'll find the amount of total fiber listed and, in some cases like on high-fiber health foods—you're likely to find the fiber broken up into its two main types: soluble and insoluble. Mounting evidence shows total fiber intake is more important than either one individually, so ignore the breakdown. Sugars normally follow fiber on the listing and, like fiber, the breakdown provided is nearly useless because different types of sugar cause nearly opposite reactions in the body. Sugar alcohols sometimes make an appearance on labels, but normally only on meal replacement bars. Currently, of the three types of carbohydrates—Fiber, Bulk Carbohydrate Sweeteners and Classical Carbs—only the total amount of fiber can be easily found.

Finally, you come to the rather dull looking protein section, which is never broken up into individual parts. Differences among protein types far outweigh the importance of knowing the total amount of sugar. The lack of any breakdown—of the different types of protein or sugar—reflects the slow, cumbersome process of getting scientific results translated into real-world information. This is shameful when dealing with food products and how they affect health. Proteins the body can't use for any important biological functions should be listed separately. While it's never a concern for everyday food products like vegetables and meat, supplements and meal replacement bars conceal large amounts of useless protein: instead of labeling as *meal replacements, imitation nutrition* may be a better description. At any rate, until resolved, the antiquated system will have to do, forcing us to rely on the total amount of protein per serving without knowing quality.

At the very bottom, outside of the boxed nutritional information, you'll find the list of ingredients. Ingredients appear in order of quantity: the food item with the highest concentration comes first. The section is actually the most difficult to understand because of exploited loopholes. Grouping items together with parentheses or brackets and tagging the collection with a strange, proprietary name gives manufacturers the ability to list ingredients in any order their creativity allows. At best, you can avoid products containing certain keywords in the list of ingredients. Further down appears a list of words to look for.

Cracking the Code

First, find out what constitutes a serving, particularly when dealing with canned and bottled beverages, and individually wrapped items like candy bars—what you might expect for a single serving is sometimes two or more. When examining the label of a product, a quick glance may reveal relatively few calories. But remember, this is the calorie count of a single serving. If the manufacturer decides a single candy bar counts as four servings, you might consume four times the amount of calories you're expecting. This goes for the number of grams of everything listed as well: four times the amount of fat, four times the amount of carbs, four times the amount of protein. Read carefully.

For fat and protein the only numbers you need to look at are those immediately to the right of the nutrient name. The example lists the total amount of fat as 7 grams (g) and total amount of protein as 5g per serving. The individual breakdowns below are relatively unimportant for The Carb Nite Solution if you follow the included menu plans; otherwise, to avoid developing a nonchalant attitude about saturated fat, try sticking to products having less than one half the total fat from saturated. Since 1.5 grams is far less than 3.5 grams (half of 7), as far as fat content is concerned, this product is a good choice.

The carbohydrate section isn't as easy. Here, look at the divisions of carbohydrates, particularly the amount of fiber. Fiber is the *only* component you need to look at, along with the total grams of carbs. Subtracting the grams of total fiber—you may have to add grams of soluble and insoluble fiber if listed separately—from the total amount of carbs gives the grams of usable carbohydrates. In the sample, 35 g total carbohydrates minus 3 g fiber gives a total of 32 g of usable carbohydrates. For this particular product, one serving completely blows your carbohydrate limit for a fat and protein day.

Turning our attention to the % Daily Value column, we find all we need to know about...absolutely nothing. The numbers listed under the % Daily Value contain useless information for any type of diet. Far too often, people make mistakes by consulting the percentages instead of the total number of grams. Misunderstanding is easy since % Daily Value numbers are normally the only elements of the label printed in bold. In reality, the percentages only distract you from meaningful information. The most common mistake occurs when reading the percentage next to carbs—in this case 12%—and confusing the percentage for the number of grams. If the product contained 12 grams total carbs per serving, one serving will not blow your daily carb limit—if you've been strict for the day. But no matter how strict, you cannot have one serving containing over 30 grams of carbs.

The ingredient list represents our last chance to eliminate a product from the diet. On any diet, and especially on Carb Nite, if you remember nothing else, remember this: avoid products with fructose, high-fructose corn syrup appearing in the first half of the ingredients. These products complicate your ability to lose body fat on any type of diet, particularly on The Carb Nite Solution. To be thorough, you can use the following list to help filter through the massive amounts of products available.

Risky Product Ingredients

Absolutely Avoid	High Avoidance	Caution
Fructose[1]	Hydrogenated Soybean Oil[2]	Hydrogenated Palm Kernel Oil[2]
Glycerin, Glycerine, Glycerol[1]	Hydrogenated Cottonseed Oil[2]	Collagen[3]
High-fructose corn syrup[1]	Hydrogenated Vegetable Oil[2]	Erythritol[1]
Hydrogenated Starch Hydrolysate (HSH) [1]	Hydrogenated Canola Oil[2]	Gelatin[3]
Isomalt[1]	Xylitol[1]	Mechanically Separated Chicken or Turkey[3]
Lactitol[1]		
Maltitol[1]		
Mannitol[1]		
Sorbitol[1]		

[1] Bulk Carbohydrate Sweetener
[2] Artificial trans-fat
[3] Poor quality protein

Net Carbs, Impact Carbs and Effective Carbs

Do not be fooled by the marketing concepts Net Carbs, Impact Carbs and Effective Carbs. Be sure to calculate the usable carbohydrates in a product by subtracting fiber from the total carb count and nothing more. Net Carbs only include carbohydrates spiking blood sugar—and consequently insulin levels—within the first hour of eating. The calculation echoes the mistake of targeting spikes for halted fat burning instead of spreading the blame correctly to low, long-lasting rises in either, which stop fat burning for several hours. As you'd expect, Net Carbs don't include fiber, which is similar to usable carbs: the difference stems from excluding Bulk Carbohydrate Sweeteners in the Net Carbs calculation. By focusing solely on blood sugar and insulin spikes while ignoring the numerous health consequences of eating Bulk Carbohydrate Sweeteners, Net Carb labels can trick you into consuming large amounts of the most devastating type of carbohydrates—devastating for fat loss and health.

Taking the second nutritional label as an example (from an Atkins Nutritionals™ Smores Flavored Bar), the usable carbs comes out to be:

Total grams of carbs		Total grams of fiber		Grams of usable carbs
26	-	11	=	15

Calculating the Net Carb count for the Smores bar, as per the instructions directly below the nutrient listing, gives:

Total grams of carbs		Total grams of fiber		Grams of glycerine		Grams of sugar alcohols		Grams of Net Carbs
26	-	11	-	8	-	4	=	3

Not only is the fiber subtracted, but two Bulk Carbohydrate Sweeteners are excluded as well: glycerol and lactitol (a sugar alcohol).

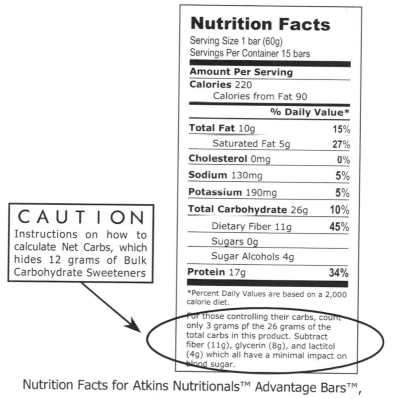

Nutrition Facts

Serving Size 1 bar (60g)
Servings Per Container 15 bars

Amount Per Serving

Calories 220
          Calories from Fat 90

% Daily Value*

Total Fat 10g — **15%**

          Saturated Fat 5g — **27%**

Cholesterol 0mg — **0%**

Sodium 130mg — **5%**

Potassium 190mg — **5%**

Total Carbohydrate 26g — **10%**

          Dietary Fiber 11g — **45%**

          Sugars 0g

          Sugar Alcohols 4g

Protein 17g — **34%**

*Percent Daily Values are based on a 2,000 calorie diet.

For those controlling their carbs, count only 3 grams pf the 26 grams of the total carbs in this product. Subtract fiber (11g), glycerin (8g), and lactitol (4g) which all have a minimal impact on blood sugar.

C A U T I O N

Instructions on how to calculate Net Carbs, which hides 12 grams of Bulk Carbohydrate Sweeteners

Nutrition Facts for Atkins Nutritionals™ Advantage Bars™, Smores Flavor

Note the difference: the Net Carb count makes you believe you can eat two, three or even four Smores bars while still easily staying under 30 grams of carbohydrates for the day. In fact, one bar contains enough Bulk Carbohydrate Sweeteners to begin the production of the carb-to-fat converting enzymes and prevents fat burning for the next few hours. Not only will you cripple your body's ability to burn any kind of fat—dietary or body—but you'll be geared up for massive fat storage come Carb Nite. Usable carbs and Net Carbs are obviously not the same: Do not confuse the two. Often, the usable grams of carbohydrates can be as much as ten times the amount of advertised Net Carbs, Impact Carbs or Effective Carbs, so ignore these proprietary terms, except when using them as a signal to avoid the product.

Planning For The Future

Your First Week

The first week of the diet, called Reorientation, is the most difficult. Contending with the temporary mental and physical sluggishness, a whole new menu, explanations to your friends and family, and curiosity about what's going to happen to your body can be draining. Being well prepared reduces the stress associated with such a radical change. Going to extraordinary efforts is unnecessary, but finding the right spices, oils and sauces to add flavor while not adding any carbohydrates challenges even the most seasoned dieter. Plan for these issues to avoid being blindsided the first day.

Regarding your first day: choose wisely. You need nine days to complete Reorientation. Figure out on what day you want the first Carb Nite to fall and start accordingly. This is the only time you'll need to plan carefully for Carb Nite, as the normal amount of flexibility allows you to choose liberally over a three day period—usually reserved for weekend dinner plans, special occasions and holidays. But for now, focus on what day you'd like that first, all-important Carb Nite.

Carb Nite Calculator	
If the first day of your diet starts on a	*Then your first Carb Nite is on a*
Sunday	Tuesday
Monday	Wednesday
Tuesday	Thursday
Wednesday	Friday
Thursday	Saturday
Friday	Sunday
Saturday	Monday

To coincide with dinner plans, let's say you decide on the following Friday for your first Carb Nite. Looking on the chart reveals a Friday Carb Nite calls for a Wednesday beginning. A Wednesday start does not allow you to eat carbs two days later—a Friday—wait until the following Friday (Wednesday, Thursday, Friday, Saturday, Sunday, Monday, Tuesday, Wednesday, Thursday *then* Friday). Going without carbs for these nine and a half days may seem like a long time; not only is it necessary, but it's also the longest period endured without the savory taste of bread.

Getting Started

Insuring success on any plan takes preparation. Deciding on Friday for your first Carb Nite, you're unlikely to wake up on Wednesday of some random week and say, "I'll go ahead and start my first nine days of The Carb Nite Solution today." Planning and a little rearranging need to take place first. Begin by cleaning out the cabinets and refrigerator. Get rid of any out-of-date products or those carb-containing products going out of date within the next nine days. Common items include milk, soft cheese, yogurt, bread, fruits, vegetables and left-overs from dinners containing pasta, noodles or rice. If still fresh, try enjoying the carb dishes one last time—well, the last time for a few days—as opposed to just throwing them out.

Next, go through your kitchen cabinets and rid the cupboards of any opened boxes of breakfast cereal, potato chips, cookies, candy or anything else tempting fate—snacking on carbs is easy when you've got cabinets full of opened packages calling your name. Move any products with large amounts of high-fructose corn syrup out of the house, as these can completely destroy even the best dieting efforts. High-fructose corn syrup is the one thing to always avoid even on Carb Nite. For the same reason—high amounts of fructose—fruit juices and soft drinks also need to go. Check any prepackaged baked goods like muffins—high-fructose corn syrup may be one of the top ingredients.

Now it's off to the grocery store to insure an ample source of quality fat and protein for the week. You should consult the list of acceptable products in the Food Lists section and also look at a weekly meal planner to assess the items you might need. Also, take the time to get acquainted with your grocery store by glancing at nutrition labels as you travel through the aisles. Remember, avoid products with Net Carb, Effective Carb and Impact Carb labels: the items most likely contain large amounts of sugar alcohols—another Bulk Carbohydrate Sweetener—which fatten you up on any type of diet.

Sample Grocery List for a
Fat and Protein Day

Date //15/05 _Grocery List_ Page #

Carb Countdown Chocolate Milk

DHA-Fortified Eggs (1 dozen)

Pepperoni

1 lb Smoked Turkey

Jack Cheese

Mozzarella Cheese Sticks

Pumpkin Seeds

Mustard

Pork Rinds

1 lb Ground Beef

Almond Oil

Flaxseed Oil

2 Ham Steaks

Snapple Diet Lime Green Tea

You're home from shopping, the groceries are put away and there's time for some meal selection. Spending the day home makes things easier, since preparing meals can be done on the fly. Otherwise, plan on packing a few meals until you familiarize yourself with the menus of local restaurants and their ingredients.

At first, the difficulty in eating away from home may seem challenging, but you'll soon find selecting food for fat and protein days is remarkably easy—especially compared with counting calories—until then, bring a few items everyday. Luckily, you'll find yourself preparing and packing little. Most people only carry enough food for one full meal and some snacks like pumpkin seeds or cheese sticks, and sometimes, even a *few* almonds. Be creative when planning: pepperoni slices, prepackaged lunch meat, sliced cheese, pork rinds and mustard, cottage cheese...well, maybe there's not much to be creative with, so bring convenient, satisfying, enjoyable foods. Travel with plenty of food during Reorientation (the first nine days of The Carb Nite Solution), even if some accompanies you home. Hunger control is important.

Reorientation is a time to change your habits and find a new routine. It takes a little time to discover tasty snack items that satisfy hunger, are easy to prepare and carry, and that you like. Most people don't consider the importance of enjoying food as much as possible. The sauce recipes in the Recipes section help season and spice up common, dull items like cheese and meat—and if you don't think cheese is dull, wait until the first month is over. Mustard is another lifesaver because the number of phenomenal tasting, specialty mustards seems to grow monthly. And most mustards maintain zero-carb status. Watch out for honey mustards though, which nearly all contain sugar.

Use these first nine days to explore the selection of foods and availability of items from the provided Food Lists. Do not, however, use these first nine days as a time to experiment with unknown foods. Stick as closely as possible to the tried and true selections that are nearly 100% safe. These include ground beef, eggs, hard cheeses, pepperoni, salami, heavy cream, olive oil, bacon, pork chops, chicken breasts and other meats, cheeses and oils. Don't forget spinach, sprouts and celery, all of which are 100% safe for fat and protein days because of fiber content. Hot peppers like jalapenos, banana peppers and wax peppers are also safe, not to mention effective at spicing things up.

Reorientation is not just about food. Your first nine days encompass reorienting thoughts and attitudes as much as hormones and enzymes. For the better part of the last 50 years we've been force-fed this notion that low-fat equals healthy, or conversely, dietary fat means death. The research reassures us at every point along the way: dietary fat is not the culprit, but a long uninterrupted period of overeating carbohydrates and fat is; especially with high levels of saturated and trans-fat in the mix. Our repulsion to bacon and eggs, or any fat-rich meal is a purely conditioned response; in this case, one unfairly forced on us. You'll find many unfounded, though still commonly held perceptions as you venture into the world of power-dieting.

Instances of myths are closer than you may realize. For example, consider three different meals. The first consists of a lean baked chicken breast, brown rice, broccoli and cooked carrots, all seasoned to taste without the use of oils or butter making for an extremely low-fat meal. Next: a plate of spaghetti with marinara sauce and whole grain bread with olive oil for dipping. Finally we're faced with a filet mignon, cooked to your preference, served with a cup of coffee with a few tablespoons of heavy whipping cream added for flavor. Of the three, which is the healthiest?

The first meal raises insulin levels, keeping them elevated for a few hours, while at the same time raising triglyceride levels—a symptom of Syndrome X. Fat storage, prevention of body fat burning and an increase in heart attack risk all result. The second meal, on the other hand, lowers heart attack risk but causes noteworthy body fat gain because of the mixture of an abundance of carbohydrates and olive oil, which contains fat cells' favorite type of fat to store. The last meal boosts metabolism, accelerates fat burning and lowers triglyceride levels, thus preventing fat storage, promoting fat burning and lowering your risk of heart attack. Do you still think lower fat meals are always healthier?

For those worried about eating too much meat, particularly red meat, here's another riddle. Who's healthier: a vegetarian who never eats animal meat or the average health conscious person who eats red meat at least weekly? Both have the same life expectancy, both have low cholesterol levels, both have the same incidence rates of various cancers, but one suffers an increased risk of stroke—the vegetarian. Nevertheless, the majority of people surveyed believe vegetarians are the healthiest among us. Another myth we've lived by for too long.

Planning for Carb Nite

Carb Nite, the veritable free-for-all, takes only minor planning.

1. Avoid soft drinks and fruit juices. The high concentrations of fructose in these items make you fat and fail to create any of the beneficial hormonal responses, regardless of how much you consume. If you're dying for a glass of orange juice on Carb Nite, try eating an orange or two.

2. Try starting Carb Nite off with a full meal including lean meat and plenty of starches like bread, pasta, rice or potatoes—the Classical Carbs. The importance of protein on Carb Nite rivals that of the carbohydrates. Protein helps create a sense of fullness and mental, Prozac®-like ease. This is where restaurants come in handy. *Restaurant*, as used here, means a decent, sit-down style of dining, not fast food like McDonald's®, Burger King® or Wendy's®—these can actually be more useful in an emergency on fat and protein days than on a Carb Nite.

3. Make sure to treat yourself to bread, pasta, pie, cobbler, cookies and other bakery items like donuts as the night continues. Eating sweets is a good thing but go for the specialty or, better yet, homemade versions of confectionaries, as many mass-marketed items contain large amounts of trans-fats and high-fructose corn syrup. If you need a candy bar, instead try some dark or bittersweet chocolate.

4. Because of the potential body fat gain, try to make the first meal or snack of the night lower in fat, but do not worry about going extremely low-fat. Choose chicken over beef, salmon over sausage. As the evening unfolds, don't feel like you can't have some donuts, a piece of cheesecake or a helping of peach cobbler—indulge.

5. Drink plenty of water and while you're at it, eat a banana or two. Your body is going to store some of those carbs in your muscles along with a lot of water. Make sure to drink plenty of fluids to avoid muscle cramping. Cramping can also result from mineral imbalances, so try eating foods high in potassium and calcium like fat-free milk, yogurt and bananas.

These are just guidelines, as nothing's set in stone for Carb Nite. The guidelines do, however, help you to achieve the maximum hormonal benefits while minimizing or completely avoiding any downside. As we know, high levels of insulin from eating sugary foods prevent fat burning and promote fat storage. But dietary fat takes roughly six hours after a meal before being available for storage and, since insulin levels drop within an hour or two of eating, you likely to avoid the possibility of adding body fat from a fatty meal on Carb Nite. So relax when deciding between cheesecake and low-fat yogurt on Carb Nite—choose what you love.

The most important factor on Carb Nite is eating plenty of Classical Carbs while avoiding Bulk Carbohydrate Sweeteners—a task you'll find surprisingly easy. And I don't care if you've been craving a large salad all day: order the pasta with meatballs or meatloaf and mashed potatoes instead. Save the salad for after dinner salad if you're still interested. The meals you normally think of as heavy and fattening are the ones that help you lose the most weight on Carb Nite. Live a little.

What To Expect

Reorientation

The first nine days reorient the body, weaning you from carbohydrates while improving fat burning efficiency. A surprisingly complex set of interactions take place for what seems like such a simple change in diet: mainly carbs to mainly fat. For those who care, the following detail helps demystify the experience.

Days 1 Through 5

A

- Carbohydrate stores are wiped out. The body still burns carbs but waning dietary levels prevent stores from being replenished. Carb stores dwindle to near nothing within about three days. Storing carbs also requires the storage of three-times as much water. As the carbs go, so will excess water. On any type of a low-carb diet, almost 80% of the initial weight loss—which can be up to 20 lbs—is from the loss of carbohydrate stores and water.

B

- While carb stores deplete, the body stops making the carb-to-fat converting enzymes. This makes it nearly impossible to store excess dietary carbohydrates as body fat.

C

- The body begins transforming fats into special molecules called ketones needed by the brain for energy when carb

77

levels fall. Full ketone production takes three to four days.

Days 4 Through 9

- After levels of stored carbs reach a minimum, the brain begins transitioning to ketones for energy. This natural and safe process takes another 3 to 4 days, during which many suffer from a mental dullness and apparent physical lethargy. This rapidly ends once the brain shifts gears.

During the first three days while carb stores are wearing away, the possibility to store some fat still exists, so don't overeat, but do control hunger. For the next month, water loss is greater before returning to normal. In essence, expect to experience some sluggishness—both mental and physical—a little dehydration, and, on average, a loss of anywhere from two to ten pounds depending on your previous diet. Make it a habit to drink plenty of water and realize you're not going to be as quick witted or footed.

Carb Nite

The tenth morning starts with ease, having etched carbs almost completely from your diet and completing Reorientation. But you'll no longer need to resist the lure of sweets, and of all things, vegetables—you'll reunite in a few hours. As dreamy as thoughts of gingerbread men and jelly beans may be, your body's got a few more surprises in store.

Withholding carbs from the body causes a carb-rebound. Called carb-loading by athletes, the reintroduction of carbs for the evening amasses a large store—not of fat, but of sugar. The body still craves those quick-burning carbs. Anticipating another carb-free stint, Carb Nite drives the body to store extra amounts of sugar in your muscles, among other places. The body continues burning fat while you're eating the carbs and your body will not switch back to carbs as its main energy source after just one evening of—enthusiastic—carb feeding. Surprisingly, the carb-frenzy actually increases fat burning for a few days.

The boost in fat burning and jolt of carbs ignites metabolism on Carb Nite. Accompanying the excess combustion, an elevated body temperature might be a bit of a surprise. Concern is unwarranted: because of the increase in metabolism, a lot of the food is wasted as heat. This can make things a little warmer than normal at bedtime. Maybe you'll want to sleep with the covers off.

Along with acting as a giant carb-sponge, your body acts like a real sponge as well, soaking up three grams of water for every gram of stored carbs. Failing to drink enough water may provoke some muscle cramping due to slight dehydration. Drinking plenty of water and eating mineral rich foods, like bananas, helps prevent cramping.

The Day After Carb Nite

Pay close attention: You're going to be storing some of the carbs and water after every Carb Nite. If you want to feel the pangs of disappointment, weigh yourself the morning after

Carb Nite. You'll feel betrayed as you view the increase in your weight from as recently as the morning before Carb Nite. Don't panic. The excess weight comes completely from stored carbs and water—you did not get fatter overnight. It's simply not possible. The more you eat, the warmer you get and that's about it.

Therefore, the morning after Carb Nite might have you feeling and looking a little softer in the mirror. Don't worry: the extra weight fades in a day or two. Return to eating less than 30 grams of carbs per day and in a couple of days you'll notice new contours, smaller bulges and looser pants.

The End

Is there something wrong here? The End? You don't end a diet. Do you?

✧✧✧

Power-dieting is a short-term proposition—that is, if you consider up to six months short-term—thus, at some point it must end, if only for a brief time. With the end of any diet comes the fear of regaining the lost weight, which traumatizes even the most stolid. What you don't need to fear on The Carb Nite Solution is regaining body fat, but as for a little weight...

Just like on Carb Nite, the body has a carb-rebound when switching back to a carb-laden diet. A little bloating and weight gain from the storage of carbs and water is unavoidable when stopping an ultralow-carb diet by reintroducing carbs. Actually, you will gain some weight, but from carbohydrate and water storage—you will not automatically gain the fat back on a normal, balanced diet. Because of the carbohydrate drought, your body over-stores carbs and water by almost twice as much. Losing five pounds during Reorientation may be countered by a gain of ten pounds during your first week off. Again, this is not fat. Within the second week off, the body returns to normal storage levels and you'll be back to holding five extra pounds of carbs and water—five extra pounds that you're stuck with for as long as you eat carbs. Nevertheless, avoiding or softening this carb-rebound by reintroducing carbs slowly may be more palatable. You may avoid the double-storage problem, but avoiding those extra five pounds—or however much you normally hold—is impossible. Suggestions for easing back into carbs, as opposed to jumping headfirst, can be found in the Meal Plans.

There is also good news. For those first three or four days after ending the diet, the body continues burning fat at an accelerated rate while conversion of carbs into fat remains greatly limited. Designed to take full advantage of these four days of accelerated fat burning, the Transition Meal Plan also undermines the double-storage problem involving carbohydrates and water. Again, choosing to use the four-day transition diet is completely up to you, as the advantage is primarily a psychological one.

The Long Term

You've completed your first round of fat stripping. Svelte, slender, slim, trim, tight, toned, ripped and chiseled will all find their way into conversations about how fantastic you look, but maybe not quite yet. Even though you're fitting into clothes you were ready to ship off to charity, and friends are envious, your final destination may require a few more cycles of dieting. Take a month or two off and allow your body some recovery time from the extremes of power-dieting. Given enough rest in between, you can continue to use the Carb Nite Solution as many times as you need to reach your goals and maintain them.

The power and beauty of this diet is the limited ability to regain fat. You've tricked your hormones into believing you were never on a diet and your fat cells were confused enough to think they were full when they were actually empty, hopefully prompting many to self-destruct—a process known as *apoptosis*. Therefore, the normal fat-rebound effect from ending The Carb Nite Solution is nearly non-existent compared with all other diets. You can use many different dieting strategies to stabilize your weight and further improve health until, or if, you decide on another cycle. You might just end up returning to your old dietary habits. But make no mistake about it, if gluttony runs high—you consistently overeat—you will regain fat.

Final Touches

Supplementation and Enhancements

As with most things in life, there's room for improving The Carb Nite Solution. Some measures are necessary, most are optional, but all are minor. Some are strictly for those wanting to extract everything possible from their time spent dieting— both the amount of fat lost and the amount of health gained. For all these reasons, the following list of supplements with descriptions and how-to's can help you get the most from your dieting experience.

- **Multivitamin and Mineral:** A multivitamin is a necessity on this diet. The lack of variety in your food choices won't always provide the required amounts of essential vitamins and minerals. You're better off with a less potent, balanced vitamin tablet like Centrum®, which may be worth taking twice per day with meals—one in the morning and one in the afternoon. Don't skip your multivitamin.

- **Psyllium Fiber:** Psyllium fiber is the main ingredient in products like Metamucil® and Colon Cleanse®. It's a naturally occurring fiber that increases regularity by both helping things pass through, as well as keeping things from making a hasty exit. A dosage of one to two teaspoons with at least half of your daily meals is a good idea. Just mix with a glass of water or other carb-less beverage and drink.

Be careful when buying psyllium fiber supplements because many contain several grams of sugar for flavoring. Stick with either pure psyllium fiber (Colon Cleanse) or the flavored, sugar-free supplements (Sugar-Free, Orange Flavored Metamucil).

- **Omega-3 Capsules:** These supplemental oils usually come in a gel-covered pill and are made from fish oil. The recommended dosage is one to three servings per day. They contain the essential fats the body needs for proper health. The vast majority of modern diets are severely deficient in these fats and this is an opportunity to correct the omega-fat imbalance.

- **Caffeine:** Caffeine has received a bad rap over the years for various reasons, but the scientific literature shows it's unjustified. Caffeine's blamed for cortisol release, but the research is inconclusive and only shows that in stressful situations—like test-taking—caffeine can cause a rise in cortisol levels. But, for most people, just the thought of taking a test raises cortisol levels. Caffeine's also recently been blamed for causing insulin release; this is conclusively false. Only when caffeine is ingested with carbs will it increase the amount of insulin released. Caffeine ingested alone or with fat and protein fails to raise insulin levels. Because it's a stimulant, caffeine fights off periods of sluggishness, especially those experienced during Reorientation, but you should strongly consider using caffeine on your fat and protein days because of its potent body fat burning ability.

- **Whey Protein Isolate:** Of all the protein choices available— beef, chicken, fish—your best choice comes from milk. The only problem is that you can't get whey protein from drinking milk. Both conventional and online health food stores carry whey protein isolate in bulk powders, which is your only available dietary source. Be sure to search for isolates and not concentrates—isolates are normally free of carbohydrates. Also, pre-made whey protein drinks are pasteurized and, therefore, no longer contain whey proteins.

- **Flaxseed Oil:** Just like omega-3 capsules, flaxseed oil contains essential fats that the diet normally lacks. It's easily added to a diet consisting of mostly fat and protein.

- **Intense Sweeteners:** Items sweetened with intense sweeteners—often artificial—are normally carbohydrate free. You should use these to your advantage whenever you feel your sweet-tooth acting up. Proceed cautiously: for reasons unknown, packets of artificial sweeteners contain carbohydrate fillers. So you should use packets in your coffee, tea or other beverages sparingly. Because it can be purchased in pure form, white stevia powder—the only naturally occurring intense sweetener—should top your list of preferred sweeteners while on The Carb Nite Solution.

- **Meal Timing:** Although deciding how many meals to eat per day is a matter of preference, if you're concerned about getting the maximum health benefits, the timing is not. The number of meals per day doesn't affect anything, but if you can manage to eat each meal at roughly the same time everyday, then you are less likely to develop insulin resistance, a pre-requisite for diabetes. Eating breakfast at 7 A.M., lunch at noon and dinner at 6 P.M. daily—or whatever times you prefer—fights off one of the most common and debilitating diseases in the Western world. Consequently, it's not how often you eat nor how many meals you eat. Insuring regular daily meal times is the important factor. But you still won't lose weight any faster.

Things to Avoid

Just as there are items you can use to enhance the diet, there are also items to ruin it. This list is much shorter.

- **Alcohol:** Avoid alcohol at all costs during your fat and protein days. No matter what advertisers imply, low-carb and even no-carb alcoholic beverages prevent your body from burning fat. Alcohol is often mentioned as having more calories than carbohydrates; this, however, is not the problem. Alcohol is the preferred fuel for the body. When there's alcohol in your system, everything else gets stored until *all* the alcohol burns off or flushes out. So a glass of no-carb vodka with your evening steak guarantees a net increase in body fat—probably not what you intended. Even Carb Nite is not a safe haven for alcohol drinkers. Drinking too much on Carb Nite causes the same problems, but worse: you lose the hormonal benefits normally provided by Carb Nite. One glass of wine on Carb Nite is fine; two is pushing it; three and you might as well kiss your fat loss for the week good-bye.

- **Bulk Carbohydrate Sweeteners:** You're probably sick of hearing about the evils of eating bulk carbohydrate sweeteners. Just remember to exercise restraint with food and beverages like prepackaged bakery items, soft drinks and fruit juice. Avoid, avoid, avoid—on or off the diet.

Included at No Extra Cost

Unlike most diets, The Carb Nite Solution includes added and highly sought after benefits. They simply come with the territory.

- **No self-torture:** You are never deprived of your favorite foods for more than a few days. Most diets force you to give up your favorite desserts or other treats. If you do happen to splurge, guilt constantly replays the death scene of your diet: all that popcorn, pudding, cake and ice cream. On this diet, you splurge weekly for success. Rather than being plagued by guilt, you're rewarded with a smaller waist size.

- **Much needed support:** This diet scheme lends itself naturally to a support group setting. If you can do this diet with a group of friends, Carb Nite is a great opportunity for a potluck or a nice dinner out to discuss your progress and share personal tips to make the diet easier and more enjoyable. There's nothing better than a Carb Nite party: all the friends and food you can enjoy.

- **Increased serotonin levels on Carb Nite:** A meal rich in carbs and protein causes a release of serotonin, the brain's feel-good hormone. You'll feel mellow all evening before enjoying a restful, refreshing night's sleep.

- **For women, reduced severity of PMS:** Every woman using this diet has reported extremely mild PMS symptoms compared with normal and an extremely mild menses as well. This is a normal consequence of a diet lower in carbohydrates since carbs actually increase estrogen levels during this time of the month, thereby increasing cycle length and severity. There have also been reports of diminished menopausal symptoms.

- **For men, stabilized testosterone levels:** Healthy levels of testosterone promote bone density, muscular development, mental performance, a sense of well-being and fat burning. As men age testosterone levels fall, but a high-fat diet fights the decline by elevating testosterone back to natural levels.

- **Mental evenness:** Eating carbohydrates produces several hormonal changes that regulate mood. When you remove carbohydrates from the diet, these hormones are able to self-regulate leaving you on a nice even keel all day, even when unable to eat on schedule.

- **Reduced flatulence:** Carbohydrate metabolism in the gut is the main source of gas production in the intestinal track. Once you remove the majority of carbohydrates entering the mouth, you also remove the majority of the gas expelled from the other end.

Cautionary Notes

There are a few drawbacks, but all easily countered:

- **Over-Heating:** Reintroducing carbs after being deprived for several days prompts the burning of nearly double the normal amount for heat production. This can lead to a slightly unsettling rise in body temperature and possible sweating on Carb Nite.

- **Constipation:** People who fail to take enough fiber and eat too much saturated fat sometimes get backed up. Including fiber throughout the day attenuate this hazard. Also, avoiding an over-abundance of saturated fat is a good recommendation if you experience trouble. Carbohydrates can stimulate bowel movements, so Carb Nite usually cleanses the system, but don't depend on this—be proactive.

- **Halitosis:** Some people experience unpleasant smelling breath on ultralow-carb diets. You might want to keep some no- or low-carb breath aids handy.

There's a final warning about Carb Nite. All aspects of The Carb Nite Solution fit together like the pieces of a puzzle; a Carb Nite can only cause the beneficial hormonal response without making you fat when used in combination with an *ultralow*-carb diet. Having regular Carb Nites on any other diet plan will only make you fat. Unfortunately, it cannot be used to enhance other types of diets, including, but not limited to, Atkins, South Beach, The Zone and The Fat Flush Program. Although many of these claim to be low-carb or carb-smart diets, they allow far too many carbohydrates for the body to react in a positive way to Carb Nite. The vast majority of the excess carbs you eat will be stored as fat. With these diets your carbohydrate stores are nearly full, your body has plenty of the carb-to-fat converting enzymes and few calories will be burned off as heat. Carb Nite with any other diet plan is a path to obesity.

This is a diet that you're either on or you're not. There's no in between. The reason for the inflexibility is a good one. Countless hours were spent poring over the research to find why the Carb Nite Solution is so powerful and to squeeze every last ounce of body-fat burning potential from it. At the time of publication of this book, there's no scientifically verifiable way to improve the approach outlined here—maybe no possible way at all. There are, however, several ways to screw it up. Most of the modifications people are inclined to make destroy not only their ability to burn body fat, but more importantly, their health. You escape sabotaging yourself by staying within the guidelines.

Parting Words

Take Something with You

Having finished reading about the most advanced, heavily researched fat loss plan available, it's time to answer a question: Is The Carb Nite Solution right for you? The answer, I hope, is a resounding "Yes", but for whatever reasons you may decide "No".

For now, if you decide The Carb Nite Solution is not for you, don't, as the saying goes, toss out the baby with the bathwater. Besides being a unified fat loss strategy, The Carb Nite Solution outlines individual tips able to improve health regardless of diet, and, in line with the goal of this book, reduce body fat. These suggestions range from supplementing with fiber to enjoying the occasional dessert. Two suggestions, however, tower above the many others.

> Supplement with omega-3 fats whenever possible:
> Reaching the proper balance between omega-3 and omega-6 fats relieves various, common problems ranging from allergies to arthritis and even reduces cancer risk. In addition to these important health benefits, increasing dietary levels of omega-3 fats restricts the storage of body fat. Try including cold-water fish, flaxseeds, flaxseed oil and supplemental capsules in your diet.

> ➤ Eliminate Bulk Carbohydrate Sweeteners:
>
> This point can never be emphasized enough. Searching for high-fructose corn syrup, fructose, glycerine and sugar alcohols among the ingredients of cookies, bakery items, soft-drinks, candy bars and, the most counterintuitive of all, nutrition bars can help you eliminate as many of these items from your diet as possible. With the average daily consumption of Bulk Carbohydrate Sweeteners reaching a staggering 30% of calories in the United States, evidence points to these carbs as a significant cause of accelerating rates of obesity, particularly among children. Once more: avoid, avoid, avoid.

Unfounded Fears

If you have read any of the latest diet books, you may be concerned about the safety of low-carb diets. The long-term safety of low-carb diets is questionable; although for at least one year, even Atkins—the highest carbohydrate version of a low-carb diet—improves every aspect of Syndrome X. In many cases, Atkins performs better than a low-fat diet. But still, several authors and experts question the long-term safety of low-carb diets, and rightfully so. They base judgments on the vast amount of research showing that a lifestyle diet consisting of large amounts of fat eaten together with high levels of carbohydrates—as allowed on an Atkins' style diet—corresponds to health problems. Authors are not, however, justified in blaming senseless, unproven things like hair loss on low-carb diets.

The various views and opinions taken on low-carb lifestyles concern us little. For one, The Carb Nite Solution is not low-carb as Atkins and others define it. The Carb Nite Solution is ultralow-carb. Every study limiting carbs to 30 grams or less per day demonstrates nothing but positive effects—more positive than a simple low-carb diet and far more positive than low-fat. Secondly, The Carb Nite Solution is not a lifestyle: it is a powerful fat-stripping tool to be used for no more than six months at a time, although you may use it repeatedly with breaks in between.   Finally, no unfounded *opinion*—by a family doctor, nutritionist or your next-door neighbor—carries as much weight as the volumes of scientific research supporting this diet. It's disappointing that so many popular diets base claims on little verified research and lots of hope. In designing The Carb Nite Solution, research was taken to the limits of the principles or documented facts, but never to the point of wishful thinking. The results are proof enough.

Now clearly, your physician may have reasons beyond mere opinion for why some of these recommendations are unsuitable for you. I strongly encourage you to consult your physician before altering your diet.

Bad Habits

During your time with The Carb Nite Solution, you learn many things: some detailed in these pages, others as enlightened afterthoughts. Muscle is precious. Dietary fat is essential to health. Carbohydrates are not. Nearly any kind of dietary fat can be healthy if you exclude carbs. And, for many, carbs underpin the excitement and variety of an enjoyable diet.

Returning to a carb-laden lifestyle seems inevitable, but upon returning avoid taking an unwelcome habit with you. Eating a substantial amount of fat, of all types, is an essential part of your success and remains healthy while on The Carb Nite Solution, but venturing beyond requires a different set of rules. When not on The Carb Nite Solution: watch your fat intake; limit sweet and creamy-smooth desserts; avoid saturated fat. Even eating too much of the "healthy" fat found in olive oil—monounsaturated—makes you fat and increases the severity of Syndrome X. So, put simply: Ratchet-back the dietary fat.

But by no means can you gorge on carbs simply because you cut back on dietary fat. Overeating carbs or fat makes people fat and overeating the two together accelerates the process in all situations other than those specifically outlined here.

A Quick Word About Exercise

Exercise is an important part of any lifestyle, health and wellness program. But this diet is not a lifestyle. This diet is designed to kick-start fat loss, not as a way to live from now through retirement and beyond. The Carb Nite Solution is a short-term tool for maximum, sustainable fat loss in a minimum of time. Where does exercise fit in?

Exercise can be used to enhance certain aspects of the diet, but it has been shown time and again that it takes over half a year before exercise impacts fat loss. Some types of exercise, like running, can even harm your health and make fat loss more difficult, particularly on an ultralow-carb diet. Therefore, for the first six-month interval of this diet, exercise is optional if your only goal is fat loss.

This is not a "get out of exercise free" card. Exercise has several benefits, making it an important addition to any lifestyle. Unfortunately, the complexity of the subject warrants its own volume. While beginning an exercise plan increases the chance of completing The Carb Nite Solution, some people have not the time nor inclination to adopt a routine at the beginning of this strategy. But, in spite of anything else you might hear or read, whatever you do, try to avoid high-intensity aerobic exercise—running, cycling, jogging, rowing—while on The Carb Nite Solution. These activities actually accelerate muscle loss and increase cortisol levels for several days, making it possible to grow new fat cells on Carb Nite. If you are performing high-intensity aerobics or are training for an endurance event, like a marathon, do not attempt to use The Carb Nite Solution unless you suspend or heavily moderate these activities for the duration of the diet. If you enjoy brisk walking or weight lifting or both, stick with these instead.

Psychology of Dieting

The Carb Nite Solution started as an asset of a limited group. Bodybuilders, and other athletes driving their bodies to extremes, rarely enjoy eating: food is a means to an end. I figured stripping carbs from the diet would discourage all but the most strict—or insane.

As The Carb Nite Solution moved beyond the bodybuilding community, something extraordinary happened. Users loved it. On the one hand, fat and protein days are easy, convenient and provide all day satisfaction. But being able to eat all the wonderful treats without the guilt, knowing Carb Nite accelerates fat loss, introduced a new world of dieting, one easily embraced by those sacrificing for most of their lives. For some, sacrificing had become so intertwined with eating that they unknowingly surrendered to depriving themselves. Before beginning The Carb Nite Solution, people tell me they love the way they eat—relieving their own doubts, as much as trying to convince me. After using this diet for only a month, they thank me for giving them the opportunity to enjoy food again.

The Carb Nite Solution can compliment the lives of everyone. Some use this plan on a three-month-on, one-month-off cycle. Others enjoy scheduling their Carb Nite Solution for October through March—wintertime for most. Their lives are more relaxed, less active, and the delectable fruits and vegetables have passed for the season. Being able to battle weight loss without feeling the need for outdoor exercise—like running, jogging and cycling—many people free up time spent on the treadmill, where few enjoy spending an hour or two. Carb Nites are planned for Halloween, Thanksgiving and Christmas, with many enjoying full carb days for the last two. Even the New Year is ushered in guilt free.

To my astonishment, this is a diet people don't want to end. People have begged to stay on longer than six months, as if contending with some spiritual leader. Keep in mind, this is a powerful tool; this is power-dieting. Your body needs a short break, as does your mind. When you've reached an undreamed of goal and the excitement to continue seems intoxicating, this is the time to take a short break. Whatever maintenance diet you choose after The Carb Nite Solution will seem like a breeze and after only a month or two of sustaining you'll begin stripping fat again with unparalleled zeal upon returning to The Carb Nite Solution.

Being Realistic

People often start diet plans expecting miracles. The blame rests mostly on diet makers and marketers pushing outrageous claims. Yet, some fault still resides with the dieter. I've been bombarded time and again with questions like, "How long is this going to take?" and "Do I really need to spend more than a month on this diet?"

Let's just be realistic. How long did it take to gain the excess fat you're trying to get rid of? Did you go from a size 4 to 14 overnight? Did your pant size increase from 30 inches to 42 inches last month? Even as a child, it took years to accumulate the excess body fat that took me 15 years to finally conquer. It took me that long because I didn't know what I know now—nobody did. With the program outlined here, I finally lost the fat in a realistic and short amount of time—over a decade of battling was ended with six months of power-dieting.

So just be honest with yourself. It took longer than a month to add the extra 30 or 40 pounds you want to lose and it's going to take longer than a month to get rid of it. It's going to take a few months and you'll possibly need to cycle on and off of The Carb Nite Solution a couple of times before reaching your desired goals. It will not, however, take years upon years. And you are not forced to diet continuously for the rest of your life, a pledge no other diet can honestly make. The only thing they can promise is to help you lose some weight while still leaving you far from your goal. Sticking with these diets to keep the weight off means never-ending self-sacrifice and frustration.

The Carb Nite Solution finally gives you control. With The Carb Nite Solution you lose body fat; you avoid a rebound effect; you can stop the diet; you can return to normal eating; you strip the fat off in a much shorter period of time than it took to put it on. In short, you can achieve the body you've dreamed of if you're willing to take just a little bit of time. Even six months will make an incredible difference in the way you look and feel. What's six months of your life compared with the six or more *years* it took to add the weight? And if you do gain back a little fat after achieving your goals, rest assured: you know how to take it back off. Best of all, this diet *requires* weekly indulgence.

✧✧✧

After all the failed attempts, years of sacrificing and near surrender, you sit back and breathe a deep sigh. Closing this final chapter in the book feels like closing a chapter in your life. Never again will you be a slave to body fat. Never again will you feel helpless. You realize this is more than just The Carb Nite Solution. This is *your* solution.

Their Carb Nite Solution

Results Are Typical

When buying a new car, computer, TV or even vacuum cleaner the opinion of others experienced with the item is invaluable. Their opinion shapes your expectations, quells your concerns and helps determine whether it's the right one for you. Diets are no different. Before test-driving one, you'd like to know if others have been successful achieving their goals—goals which you share.

But the diet and weight loss industry adds a unique twist. Diet advertising consists of testimonials and results from those who've used the plan followed by a curious phrase: *Results not typical.* My personal favorite, which represents the average claim, is an advertisement for Bill Phillips' *Eating For Life.* It goes something like, "Suzy lost 43 lbs*. You can too!" Excited? Well, there it is at the bottom of the ad in print so small as to be overlooked by anyone without a magnifying glass: **Results not typical.* If the results aren't typical, what is meant by, "You can too"? If the results aren't typical, then we most likely can't.

Breaking with tradition, here are the *typical* stories of average dieters who achieved their goals using The Carb Nite Solution.

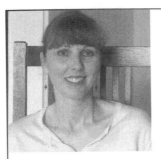

Brenda Given
Age 46
Marketing Executive

I've been a chronic dieter since my teens so I was somewhat open to trying The Carb Nite Solution, even though it was quite counter intuitive. Although I've never been overweight, I've worked hard to eat healthy and exercise in the hopes of staying lean, fit and illness free. Despite a lifetime of rigor and deprivation, my body fat percentage was always higher than it should be. I spent many years as a vegetarian and awhile as a strict vegan and still couldn't reduce my body fat. Even several hours of daily exercise and substantial resistance training didn't work as well as I expected.

After a few months on The Carb Nite Solution, however, I did see a reduction in stubborn body fat. My stomach, my thighs and my underarms shrank as a result of losing 10 pounds. My clothes fit better, I looked and felt better and best of all I didn't lose any muscle, which is increasingly difficult for me to maintain. I also experienced noticeable improvement in my early menopausal symptoms—fewer hot flashes, less cramping and lighter flows. I've never had such dramatic results from any other diet.

I now have a heightened awareness of the tremendous impact food has on the body—both positive and negative. And I have a new tool that I can use to control body fat that doesn't require a lifelong lifestyle change. It's comforting to know I have the power to keep fat at bay as I age.

Jim Given
and his cat, Sophie
Age 51
Corporate Attorney

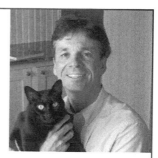

I have never been very overweight, but I have suffered from the "pound or two per year" creep since I got out of school. I used to think that this "filling out" was inevitable, until one year I found that my belly was interfering with the upward range of movement of my knees while riding my bike. I resolved to change that quickly, and did. Over three months, I lost around 30 pounds on the typical restricted-calorie diet (hitting a hard plateau there), but I lost an awful lot of muscle, too.

Five years later, after slowly regaining half the lost weight back, I tried The Carb Nite Solution. In a month, I lost fifteen pounds and a little muscle, because I inadvertently reduced calories and carbs at the same time. A year later, I thought I would try to lean down some more and lost another five pounds in a month's time without perceptible muscle loss, since I tried hard to maintain calories while controlling carbs. Now I am back to my stable, graduate weight. And I know how to stay at this weight. If I do creep up while eating normally over the year (typically during the holidays), a post-New-Year's-Day Carb Nite Solution quickly does the trick.

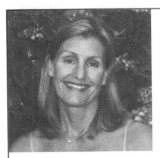

Margaret Martin
Age 49
Pilates Instructor

At first, it was hard to figure out what to eat, but after 2 weeks, it was really easy. I hadn't eaten bacon or much cheese in about 10 years before starting The Carb Nite Solution. Before long, I was looking forward to my eggs and bacon for breakfast. I found it to be very satisfying.

I could tell my blood sugar was very even and balanced on this diet compared with before because I didn't have huge cravings or mood swings. The protein shakes with fiber and flaxseed oil were the best way to stay regular and I also found red and green bell peppers to be a great source of fiber. Sometimes the food got a little dull, so I relied on the recipes (especially the Flourless Brownies) and Carb Countdown chocolate milk. I also ate out at restaurants, which was much easier than I thought. Almost every restaurant has something I can eat on fat and protein days and most places are very willing to support an ultralow-carb diet.

My Solution lasted 3 months. Shortly after the first month is when I began to feel very lean and noticed my clothes fit better. I was excited to see results so quickly. It's been eight months since I ended my diet and I still look and feel great, but I might need to go back on The Carb Nite Solution after the holidays!

Mori Taheripour
Age 33
Entrepreneur and
University Lecturer

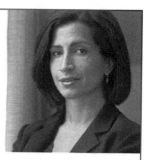

The Carb Nite Solution is great! My body was completely reshaped. My abdominal area has always been difficult to trim. But after the first ten days, and all throughout, I was leaner than I had ever been before. For the first time, I was able to see the rewards of my years of working out. I finally saw tone and muscle.

The most remarkable part of this diet was that once the first 10 days were over, I was able to look forward to my Carb Nite every weekend. For the first time, in all my life of dieting and following strict diet regimens, I did not feel deprived since I knew that I had a chance to eat my very favorite foods in just a few days!

While the first ten days without carbs seemed really daunting at first, I saw the dramatic results right away and felt more motivated every day. I was never very lethargic (except for the morning after Carb Nite when my body was trying to work through the truck-loads of food that I had managed to consume). Psyllium fiber also became my very best friend along with bell peppers. You do need a good deal of fiber to help flush out your system.

Even while traveling for work, I stayed on the diet for almost 4 months. I have actually never stuck to a diet the way I did with The Carb Nite Solution and if you can do it with a friend, it's even better. Carb Nites are so much more fun with friends!

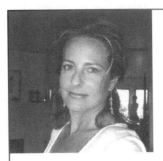

Tina Hawks

Age 34

Massage Therapist

I have never gone on a diet in my life. I've always eaten what I considered healthy and, through trial and error, ate what my body agreed with. I wasn't out of shape, but have what a lot women have trouble loosing: annoying body fat commonly called saddlebags. It didn't matter how well I ate or how hard I worked out, it never came off. Some friends were on The Carb Nite Solution and were obviously getting results. This peaked my interest and so I decided to give it a shot.

A lot of the food that's on The Carb Nite Solution I traditionally stayed clear of, so the change was hard to get use to. I was worried about that heavy, tired feeling that you get from eating a burger with french fries, but taking out the carbs completely avoided that uncomfortable, full feeling.

My first Carb Nite was a bit uncomfortable, though. I had cookies, cake, ice cream and a few other "forbidden" foods. I remember thinking, "If I get fat, I'm going to get really mad." It didn't take long before I was really enjoying my Carb Nites. I've never had so much fun with food.

When ending the diet I reached a lean 115 lbs and I felt great. I also experienced some amazing health benefits with PMS. I experienced absolutely no PMS while on the diet. If my weight ever gets a little out of control this is definitely my diet of choice to get me back on track.

Lee Agustin
Age 27
Police Officer
*picture withheld by request**

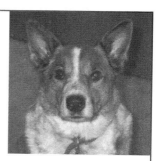

I've been weight training and dieting since I was in High School. I recently began to notice that losing weight was getting harder and my career didn't make training or dieting any easier, either.

On The Carb Nite Solution I was able to go from 220 lbs to 183 lbs in only four months. With the easy to follow dieting principles I was able to lose the weight I wanted without the cravings. The most challenging part for me was Reorientation. I was tired, lethargic, and my workouts suffered. But as I moved into the next phase of the diet these symptoms quickly went away. I know it sounds corny but, for me, losing weight and seeing immediate results was fun.

As a plus on the diet, the first area where I began to lose weight was from my waist area. I had always had a size 36-inch waist. I lost two inches on my waistline. Since then I've kept my 34-inch waistline and the weight off since I ended the diet.

---

* Pictured instead is the author's dog, Duncan, who really enjoys his fat and protein days.

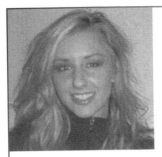

Lacy Kennedy
Age 22
Orthodontic Assistant

I'm an active woman in my twenties. My body is very important and I take pride in how I look and feel. I was recently introduced to The Carb Nite Solution and wanted to see if I could incorporate it into my daily schedule. To my surprise, it was perfect for my busy lifestyle. To my bigger surprise, in the first couple of months I could see impressive results.

As for my meals, the first ten days were my biggest adjustment. I love to snack so I learned to always have food on me to resist any temptation at the workplace.

I can still remember indulging on that first Carb Nite. It was great! After a couple of Carb Nites, they became easy to plan around. Carb Nites are nice for making plans with friends because I can eat anything I want while burning fat all night. My favorite part is indulging in foods everyone loves that are sweet and tempting. Using decadent foods to increase fat loss seems like a breakthrough for us sweet-tooth people.

Sue Dennett
Age 59
Business Owner

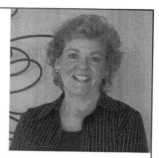

Well, the first week on The Carb Nite Solution proved to be a little difficult for me because I was so disorganized. I figured out that I needed to carry some food if I was going to be out all day and that was very different for me. I also didn't read the plan thoroughly enough and misunderstood what Carb Nite was all about: my first Carb Nite was a piece of bread at lunch. After speaking to a friend on the diet, I realized what I was doing wrong. In just a couple of weeks I learned to pack my lunch efficiently and how to have fun with my Carb Nite. From then on, it became less challenging and more rewarding. It didn't take long before it became natural.

Once I got on track, it only took a few months before I was having fun packing up my fat clothes. I never even stepped on a scale and I thought I wasn't losing any weight until I tried on clothes that I hadn't worn in years because they were too small. They all fit comfortably now and I keep fitting into older and smaller clothes. I remember going to a small party and being so excited. When I got there I said, "Guess what. These used to be tight," while I pulled at my waistline. After my fifth month I'm elated that I can take six huge bags of clothes to charity and be out there shopping for my new, slimmer self.

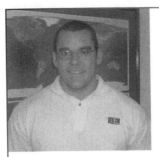

Clint Smith
Age 25
Civil Engineer

As an amateur bodybuilder, I've had great success with The Carb Nite Solution. I used the diet for my first bodybuilding competition where I took 1st place in my weight class. The diet allowed me to lose all that stubborn fat I had been carrying since I was a kid and I went to the contest super-lean.

Sometimes the diet seems difficult, but the results are real. The fact that you know you have a Carb Nite coming up also helps you stay very disciplined during the strict ultralow-carb days. Being on the diet was exciting because I could directly feel and notice the effects that it was having on my body. I never had strong hunger pains on the low carb days. The Carb Nites were always interesting because I could tell my body was burning the carbs like a furnace by the way my body temp would rise.

I have shared this diet with a couple of my friends and it has become our "Secret Weapon" when we want to strip the body fat off.

Mo Stockdale
Age 49
Independent Consultant

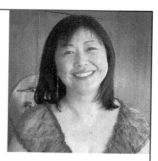

It may sound like a cliché, but The Carb Nite Solution changed my life. Every diet I had ever tried only worked for a short while since it really did not change how I looked at food. I was an admitted carb-aholic. Bread, rice, potatoes were something I could never pass up. I really didn't think I'd be able to stick with this diet, but once I was past day 2, I didn't have the cravings and it was much easier to stay on the diet. Then a miracle happened...I had much more energy! I took up West Coast Swing dancing and am now dancing 5-6 nights a week. I've gone down 5 pants sizes while on this diet and am the size I was 25 years ago. I cannot possibly be more thankful for using The Carb Nite Solution.

The Carb Nite Solution Summary

Overview

Reorientation:
For the first nine days keep carbohydrates to 30 grams or less per day—equivalent to two slices of white bread; only fiber does not count as a carbohydrate in this total. Eat enough food to keep hunger under control without worrying about counting calories.

Carb Nite™:
Day ten starts off like the previous nine days but starting at around dinner time (sometime between 4 and 6 pm) you must eat a sizable amount of carbs: spaghetti, apricots, pie, potato-chips, bread, bananas, bagels, donuts, ice-cream, cookies, cheesecake and almost anything else you've been craving. You should eat carbs for the rest of the evening—this includes all the way until bedtime and maybe even a midnight snack.

Day after your first Carb Nite™:
Go back to 30 grams or less of carbohydrates per day—the same as your first nine days.

Long Haul:
For up to six months you continue this cycle of having a Carb Nite™ at least once per week, but you must keep them at least four full days apart. For instance, if you have a Carb Nite on Friday, you cannot have your next Carb Nite any sooner than Wednesday.

Rules

1. Eat plenty of fat
2. Enjoy a *full* Carb Nite
3. Never skip Carb Nite
4. Only one Carb Nite a week

FAQs

Why a Carb Nite and not a Carb Morning or entire Carb Day?

After a high-carb meal at any point during the day—particularly breakfast—switching to an ultralow-carb meal plan has a negative impact on blood chemistry. So, you can't simply have a "carb morning"—you should finish out the day with carbohydrates. But a full day's worth of carbs potentially leads to fat gain. Being designed for the most rapid possibly fat loss while maintaining or improving health, The Carb Nite Solution does not incorporate regular "carb mornings" or "carb days". Additional reasons do, however, exist for eating carbs at night:

- After being deprived of carbs for so long, Carb Nite makes you sleepy.

- A high carb meal right before bed increases sleeping metabolism.

- Lying down helps the digestion of carbohydrates.

With that being said, having one or two full Carb Days during an entire six months of The Carb Nite Solution will not significantly slow your fat loss.

When I start Carb Nite at 4 o'clock, I have a hard time getting in a full six hours of carbs, and forget about eight. Is it possible to start my Carb Nite at lunchtime?

Yes. Just be sure to start the day without carbohydrates (a fat and protein breakfast) and stop eating carbs by 6 or 8 pm.

You say never have the next Carb Nite sooner than the fifth night after your last one. Can I just have a Carb Nite every fifth night if my schedule allows it?

You may be able to. For some, however, their bodies adapt more rapidly to The Carb Nite Solution, forcing them to end the diet sooner than planned: sometimes in less than month. A few people have succeeded while having Carb Nite every fifth night. Many more have failed by trying to attempt Carb Nite more than once per week. The risk you take by having Carb Nite more than once per week is failure. That's why I highly recommend you stick with once per week.

Why can't I just eat carbs one day then not eat them the next and go back and fourth? Won't this accomplish the same thing?

This won't accomplish the same thing, however, it can make you fat. Your body needs time to adjust after having carbohydrates and doesn't fully empty the small store of carbs until after the third or fourth day after a Carb Nite. Don't worry though: you're still burning fat while carb stores dwindle. If you eat carbs sooner than this, carbohydrate stores would remain full and you'd begin to burn less and less fat on the fat and protein days while storing more and more. As of the publication of this book, there's no known way to shorten the interval between Carb Nites without getting fat. Specifically designed studies are needed to discover if this is possible.

Can I shorten Reorientation to less than nine and a half days and by how much?

Yes. See the question below for details on how to shorten the Reorientation timeframe. As for, by how much, depends heavily on the amount of exercise you perform and type, but there is a shortest possible time. Assuming you completely exhaust carbohydrate stores the first day, which is possible, your brain still needs the next three days to build up to the efficient use of ketones, and three days are also needed for levels of the carb-to-fat converting enzymes to approach zero. So, at best, you could shorten Reorientation to four and a half days, having your first Carb Nite on the fifth night.

Is there anyway I can incorporate high-intensity cardio-vascular exercise while on The Carb Nite Solution?

Only one problem makes high-intensity cardio unsuitable for an ultralow-carb diet: at heart rates above 65% of maximum, the body exclusively burns carbs. Normally, burning carbs is an advantage, if you're eating them. But on The Carb Nite Solution, when you're not eating carbs for most of the week—which depletes stores—your body turns to the next readily available source of carbohydrates, protein. Not only will dietary protein be converted to sugar, so will your muscles. Cortisol levels also rise, staying elevated for several days making it possible to create new fat cells on Carb Nite. These scenarios run contrary to preserving muscle while burning body fat and minimizing a rebound.

If eliminating cardio is not an option for you, but you still want to use The Carb Nite Solution, there is a way to minimize the downside while still getting the maximum benefit from both the cardiovascular exercise and diet. During the first week, while your body's carb stores are nearly full, cardio is safe and can actually shorten Reorientation by a few days. Avoid the cardio for at least two days before the first Carb Nite.

After Reorientation, high-intensity aerobic work should be saved for the two to three days following a Carb Nite. If, for example, Carb Nite falls on a Friday, go cycling, running or swimming on Saturday, Sunday and even a little on Monday. High-intensity aerobics performed after this point only destroys muscle and creates an environment ripe for the birth of new fat cells.

I'm thinking of skipping Carb Nite this week to help accelerate fat loss: What do you think?

Carb Nite spikes hormones resulting in accelerated fat loss and prevents the hormonal lulls that can slow or even stop fat loss. By skipping Carb Nite for a week, hormonal levels stay depressed for a longer period of time, which means little to no fat burning. Instead of accelerating fat loss, skipping Carb Nite for a week actually slows fat loss.

Should I watch my fat intake on Carb Nite?

With your first carbs, yes you should. Not only might you store some fat, but a low-fat, high-carbohydrate Carb Nite creates the maximum hormonal benefit. As the evening wears on, don't worry so much about dietary fat content. Insulin levels—which cause fat storage when elevated—fall before the dietary fat is available for energy or storage, making it difficult to store body fat. By the time dessert rolls around, I wouldn't worry about a piece of cheesecake or a bowl of ice cream. Actually, I wouldn't worry about two pieces of cheesecake.

I really enjoy fruits and vegetables. Is it OK to have as much as I want on Carb Nite?

Be careful. High levels of insulin are the catalyst for most of the beneficial hormonal effects causing rapid and ongoing fat loss. Many fruits and vegetables are packed with fiber and normally have a low insulin index, meaning a small rise in insulin levels. Also, fructose, found in high levels in many fruits, skyrockets levels of the carb-to-fat enzymes and causes fat storage, even on Carb Nite. Therefore, limit your fruit intake to a few pieces and use fibrous vegetables, like broccoli and asparagus, to complement a meal rather than as a meal in themselves. A list of the best fruits for Carb Nite can be found in the Food Lists section.

Should I stay away from high-glycemic carbs on Carb Nite?

Quite the contrary: If anything, avoid low-glycemic carbs. See the above question for more detail.

You allow alcohol on Carb Nite but is it possible to drink too much on Carb Nite?

You can always drink too much alcohol. I would limit myself to two drinks, tops. Most people, even heavy drinkers, rarely find problem lessening their alcohol consumption. The elevated levels of serotonin caused by Carb Nite make you less likely to crave that second or third drink.

I get leg cramps from time-to-time after an indulgent Carb Nite. A friend told me to drink tonic water because it contains quinine. Will this help?

Quinine does relieve leg cramping, but the amount in tonic water is so low you'll need to drink three to six liters before reaching an effective dosage—that's around a gallon of tonic water. Diet tonic water is, however, an excellent beverage for fat and protein days, especially when combined with sugar-free syrups. See the Recipes section for an example.

What should I do if I screw up and have carbs for a couple of days in a row?

To be safe, start over with Reorientation and go from there. If this is a frequent occurrence, seek the help of a support group made up of friends, family and others on The Carb Nite Solution.

Should I worry about eating too much cheese?

It depends on what you mean by *too much*. If you're making cheese your main source of fat on the diet then, yes, you're probably eating too much cheese. Cheese contains a lot of saturated fat. Make sure you're getting plenty of monounsaturated and polyunsaturated fats as well. Don't avoid cheese, though. Dairy sources of calcium — like cheese — prove effective at enhancing fat loss. Also, cheese is a rich source of high quality protein. So, while you don't want to make cheese your main source of fat, you do want to include it as a regular staple in your diet.

Should I watch my intake of other dairy products besides cheese during the week?

Absolutely. Check the label on a carton of milk and you'll find a large amount of carbs per serving — one cup can blow half your allowance of carbs for the day. To satisfy any cravings you may have, try the dairy beverage Carb Countdown®. Carb Countdown is extremely low in carbohydrates with double the amount of protein of regular milk. Although many products with an Atkins Approved™ symbol are unsuitable for an *ultralow*-carb diet, Carb Countdown can be a useful addition to fat and protein days on The Carb Nite Solution.

Should I eat just egg whites or the entire egg while on The Carb Nite Solution?

Eat the entire egg. Compared to an entire egg, egg whites are an inferior source of protein. Also, with the availability of eggs fortified with DHA, an important omega-3 fatty acid, you have even more reason to eat the entire egg because the yolk contains these beneficial, essential fats—not the whites. Just be careful to keep track of the carbohydrates—eggs are not normally carb-free.

I read that dietary fiber may not prevent colon cancer. Is this true? If so, why do you recommend eating so much?

Research testing the preventative effects of fiber on the recurrence of colon cancer and precancerous polyps has turned up nothing. There is, however, a substantial amount of population based studies that have found a direct correlation on life-long fiber intake and a decrease in the incidence of colon cancer (actually several types of cancer) but this may point to some other life-style factor tied to fiber intake. Even though the results on colon cancer prevention are inconclusive, fiber still possesses many benefits apart from protective effects on the colon, such as the prevention of constipation. Fiber should be included in any health-conscience diet.

For Carb Nite, you say it's OK to eat through the night, but on fat and protein days should I make sure to stop eating at least three hours before bedtime?

If anything, you should eat right before bedtime. Despite conventional wisdom, eating right before bedtime is far more effective for health and fat loss—but not necessarily for weight loss—than avoiding late-evening meals. Although many fitness experts speak as though years of science have been spent dealing with this question, I could only locate one study. Participants (all women) eating a low-calorie diet were separated into two groups. Group 1 ate the majority of their calories at breakfast and very little during the rest of the day. Group 2 ate very little all day, while eating the vast majority of their calories right before bedtime. Both groups ate the same number of calories per day. The initial results harmonize with the establishment—the women who ate the majority of their calories first thing in the morning lost more *weight* than those eating just before bedtime. But when researchers determined what was lost, either muscle or fat, the results are shockingly different. Those eating most of their calories first thing in the morning lost more muscle and less body fat—muscle weighs more than fat. The late-day eaters, by contrast, actually lost more body fat and kept more muscle, becoming far healthier than their early-morning counterparts: yet another nearly universal myth with potentially harmful effects on health. Also contrary to current popular thinking, quality of sleep is not affected by eating right before bed.

Should I use keto-sticks to track my fat loss progress?

There's no need to purchase any type of urinary ketone measuring device—they tell you nothing important. Since the body produces ketones from fat—either dietary or body— during a low-carb diet, reasoning that urinary ketone levels might indicate fat loss seems plausible. Research testing this theory shows the contrary: urinary ketone levels do not indicate the rate of body fat loss. Additionally, some people expel near zero levels of urinary ketones on a low-carb diet while still losing substantial amounts of body fat.

I feel like my weight loss has started to slow down. Should I cut calories?

Absolutely not. First, be sure the bathroom scale is not your only measure of progress—scales are deceiving. Secondly, an ultralow-carb diet causes only subtle changes in the body mimicking starvation while still allowing you to eat ample amounts of food. This preserves muscle while still shedding unwanted body fat. Cutting calories changes the situation from mimicking starvation to being starvation—as far as the body is concerned. At this point, you will destroy the majority of benefits from using The Carb Nite Solution. Fat loss slows even more, muscle wastes away, cortisol levels rise and new fat cells may begin growing. Just keep in mind that as you lose body fat it gets harder to lose even more, so your progress will slow, even on The Carb Nite Solution.

You dismiss cutting calories as an effective weight loss strategy, but I noticed the included meal plans could be considered low-calorie for some people. Is The Carb Nite Solution just a low-calorie diet in disguise?

The included meal plans form the groundwork for your daily nutritional needs and I assume between-meal snacking and additional food items will accompany the scheduled meals; by no means are you expected to strictly adhere to meal plans. But, even if this is the case and there's minimal snacking, the average Carb Nite for dieters consists of a large number of calories—a whole day's worth of calories is eaten in a single night. Therefore, when considering total weekly calories, it becomes difficult to consider The Carb Nite Solution a low-calorie diet.

I've been on the diet for about two months now and I'm starting to get headaches. I'm a little concerned. Should I quit?

If you're experiencing dull, recurrent headaches while using The Carb Nite Solution and this is uncommon for you, the problem is probably too little dietary fat. The first rule for The Carb Nite Solution is to eat plenty of fat. If you eat too little fat and too much protein, you end up burning protein for energy, which accelerates muscle loss and stops fat loss. The headaches stem from 1) elevated, but constantly low blood sugar levels, leaving your brain too little energy to function properly and 2) a buildup of excess waste products from the inefficient burning of protein. Use the tools for balancing meals (food scoring and food score calculator) or one of the balanced meal plans for a week and the headaches will soon fade.

When I end The Carb Nite Solution won't I just gain all the fat back that I lost if I eat carbohydrates again?

No, you won't. There's a lot of confusing statements out there telling consumers they'll just gain all the weight back once they stop a low-carb diet. You will automatically gain some weight back, but not body fat. Like any low-carb plan, you will store an excess of carbohydrates and water when you stop the diet, but only for about a week. This is not fat gain— it's mostly water. You'll notice a slightly similar effect every morning after Carb Nite, which fades within a day or two. Even though one or two carb meals can trigger the production of carb-to-fat enzymes, the entire system can take up to 20 days before it's back to normal and ready for high-capacity conversion of carbs into fat. So, overeating carbs a little bit won't matter too much for the first week off the diet. Unless you're overeating carbs with a lot of fat—that will make you fat.

South Beach, *The Abs Diet* and *The 3-Hour Diet* all promise special techniques for losing stomach fat first. How does The Carb Nite Solution compare?

This is one claim all three diets make honestly. These three diets do cause the loss of abdominal fat first—as does every single weight reducing diet ever conceived. Losing fat from the abdominal area before thinning begins elsewhere is a consequence of losing weight, regardless of method. Since The Carb Nite Solution is designed to produce the most rapid possible fat loss, you will notice a swift loss of abdominal fat.

Is The Carb Nite Solution safe for children?

There's over 80 years of research involving the use of ultralow-carb diets with epileptic children. Otherwise promoting normal health, ultralow-carb diets may slow physical growth at young ages. For this reason, maintaining a balanced diet including whole grains, fruits and vegetables more aptly suits the nutritional needs of children. For teenagers, however, The Carb Nite Solution can be highly effective.

My doctor told me to eat a low-fat diet because dietary fat irritates my acid-reflux. Does this mean I can't use The Carb Nite Solution?

You should check with your physician in case you suffer from more than common acid-reflux. Assuming no other ailments, research conclusively shows that it doesn't matter what the meal is made of—carbohydrate, protein or fat—an excessive volume of food irritates acid-reflux. The Carb Nite Solution actually helps with your condition since meals on fat and protein days consist of small quantities of food—small because fat has such a high calorie count.

You talk about saving as much muscle as possible when using The Carb Nite Solution. As a woman, I don't really want to be muscular. Will this result from using The Carb Nite Solution?

Absolutely not. Saving muscle has little to do with achieving a muscular—or overly muscular—physique unless you're taking other steps to achieve the goal, like weightlifting. Sparing muscle tissue not only refers to preserving biceps, pecs and glutes, but also your internal organs. Most of your internal organs are made of lean tissue. Other diets not only cause the destruction of the muscles you see, but of the vital organs you need for survival. So, sparing as much muscle and lean tissue as possible while reducing body weight will not make you look like a competitive bodybuilder—it only improves your health.

The Carb Nite Solution makes it seem like desserts and sweets are actually healthy. Is it OK to make cheesecake a regular part of my diet when I'm not using The Carb Nite Solution?

On The Carb Nite Solution—particularly on Carb Nite—cheesecake can help accelerate fat loss for the upcoming week. But simply because a food item accelerates fat loss on The Carb Nite Solution does not make it healthy for other types of diets. This goes for nearly all high-calorie, high-carbohydrate, high-fat foods. Only because of the special chemical and hormonal situation created during the week does eating cheesecake, cobbler or other confectionaries cause a response resulting in healthy changes, particularly when eaten later during the evening. On any other diet plan, these types of food make you fat and deteriorate your health.

Food Lists

Usage

A difficulty finding the right foods usually accompanies starting any new diet plan. Hours upon hours can be wasted in the grocery store and bookstore researching the foods best suited to your new plan. The following lists simplify the process by providing hundreds of easy to find grocery items.

Along with important information, like serving size and grams of fiber, usable carbohydrates, fat and protein, the lists contain a score for each food, helping you to balance your meals without tedious calculations. The five Food Scores are F+, F, N, P and P+. F stands for fat, N for neutral and P for protein. Balancing between fat and protein at each meal is simple: if you decide on an F (or F+) food for a meal—breakfast, lunch, dinner or snacks—simply try to find a P (or P+) food to accompany it and vice versa. Add neutral foods to any meal or make them a meal in them self without needing complimentary items.

Finally, foods marked in gray contain carbohydrates; otherwise, they're carb-free.

Safe Foods on Fat and Protein Days

	Serving Size	Usable Carbs (g)	Fiber (g)	Fat (g)	Protein (g)	Score
Vegetables						
Alfalfa Sprouts	1 cup	0	1	0	1	P+
Arugula, fresh	1/2 cup	0	1	0	0	N
Asparagus, raw	4 spears	0	1	0	2	P+
Baby Spinach	3 cups	0	2	0	2	P+
Celery	2 stalks	0	2	0	1	P+
Green Olives	1 oz	0	1	4	0	F+
Kimchee	1/2 cup	0	4	0	2	P+
Pimientos	1 tsp	0	0	0	0	N
Romaine Lettuce, shredded	1 cup	0	1	0	0	N
Watercress, raw	1 cup	0	0	0	1	P+
Artichoke Hearts, marinated	2 pieces	1	1	5	0	F+
Banana Pepper	1 medium	1	2	0	1	P+
Bibb Lettuce, shredded	1 cup	1	1	0	1	P+
Boston Lettuce, shredded	1 cup	1	1	0	1	P+
Cauliflower, cooked	1/2 cup	1	2	0	1	P+

Vegetables

	Serving Size	Usable Carbs (g)	Fiber (g)	Fat (g)	Protein (g)	Score
Chinese Broccoli	1 cup	1	2	1	1	N
Garlic	1 clove	1	0	0	0	N
Green Onion	3 stalks	1	1	0	0	N
Hearts of Palm, canned	1/2 cup	1	2	0	2	P+
Iceberg Lettuce, shredded	1 cup	1	1	0	0	N
Jalapeno	1/2 cup	1	1	0	0	N
Pickle, dill	1 spear	1	0	0	0	N
Radicchio, raw shredded	1 cup	1	0	0	0	N
Rhubarb, raw	1 stalk	1	1	0	0	N
Sauerkraut	1/2 cup	1	2	0	0	N
Bamboo Shoots, canned	1 cup	2	2	0	2	P+
Cabbage, shredded	1 cup	2	2	0	0	N
Zucchini	1/2 cup	2	1	0	0	N
Bell Pepper, green	1 medium	3	2	0	0	N
Bell Pepper, red	1 small	3	1	0	0	N
Broccoli	1 stalk	3	3	0	2	P+
Green Beans	1/2 cup	3	2	0	1	P+
Turnips, cooked	1/2 cup	3	2	0	0	N
Yellow Beans	1/2 cup	3	2	0	2	P+

Mushrooms

	Serving Size	Usable Carbs (g)	Fiber (g)	Fat (g)	Protein (g)	Score
Chanterelle	3.5 oz	0	6	0	2	P+
Enoki	1 medium	0	1	0	0	N
Morel	3.5 oz	0	7	0	2	P+

Nuts and Seeds

	Serving Size	Usable Carbs (g)	Fiber (g)	Fat (g)	Protein (g)	Score
Flax Seeds	1 tbsp	0	3	4	2	F
Pumpkin Seeds, hulled	1/4 cup	0	1	15	11	F
Hazelnuts, raw	15 nuts	1	2	13	3	F+
Macadamia, roasted	12 nuts	1	2	22	2	F+
Pecans	20 nuts	1	3	20	3	F+
Almonds	22 nuts	2	3	15	6	F+
Pistachios	30 nuts	3	2	10	5	F

Soups

	Serving Size	Usable Carbs (g)	Fiber (g)	Fat (g)	Protein (g)	Score
Beef Broth, canned	1 cup	0	0	1	3	P
Swanson®						
Chicken Broth, 99% fat free	1 cup	0	0	0	1	P+
Chicken Bouillon Cube, prepared	1 cup	1	0	1	1	N
Beef Bouillon Cube, prepared	1 cup	2	0	1	1	N

	Serving Size	Usable Carbs (g)	Fiber (g)	Fat (g)	Protein (g)	Score
Breads						
La Tortilla Factory™						
Whole Wheat Low-Carb/Low-fat Tortillas Original Flavor	1 Tortilla	3	8	2	5	P
Whole Wheat Low-Carb/Low-fat Tortillas Garlic & Herb	1 Tortilla	3	8	2	5	P

Cheeses

	Serving Size	Usable Carbs (g)	Fiber (g)	Fat (g)	Protein (g)	Score
Beaufort	1 oz	0	0	9	8	F
Brie	1 oz	0	0	8	6	F
Cantal	1 oz	0	0	9	7	F
Chabichou	1 oz	0	0	8	6	F
Chaource	1 oz	0	0	7	5	F
Cheddar	1 oz	0	0	9	7	F
Comte	1 oz	0	0	9	8	F
Derby	1 oz	0	0	10	7	F
Edam	1 oz	0	0	8	7	F
Fontina	1 oz	0	0	9	7	F
Goat, hard	1 oz	0	0	10	9	F
Goat, semisoft	1 oz	0	0	8	6	F
Goat, soft	1 oz	0	0	6	5	F

Cheeses

	Serving Size	Usable Carbs (g)	Fiber (g)	Fat (g)	Protein (g)	Score
Gorgonzola	1 oz	0	0	9	5	F
Gruyere	1 oz	0	0	9	8	F
Jarlsberg	1 oz	0	0	7	7	N
Monterey Jack	1 oz	0	0	8	7	F
Muenster	1 oz	0	0	8	7	F
Stilton, blue	1 oz	0	0	10	7	F
Stilton, white	1 oz	0	0	9	6	F
Triple Crème	1 oz	0	0	11	3	F+
Yogurt	1 oz	0	0	7	6	F
Blue	1 oz	1	0	8	6	F
Caraway	1 oz	1	0	8	7	F
Cheshire	1 oz	1	0	9	7	F
Colby	1 oz	1	0	9	7	F
Cream Cheese	1 oz	1	0	10	2	F+
Feta	1 oz	1	0	6	4	F
Gouda	1 oz	1	0	8	7	F
Mozzarella	1 oz	1	0	7	6	F
Neufchatel	1 oz	1	0	7	3	F+
Parmesan	1 oz	1	0	8	11	N
Provolone	1 oz	1	0	7	7	N
Ricotta, Whole Milk	1 oz	1	0	4	3	F

	Serving Size	Usable Carbs (g)	Fiber (g)	Fat (g)	Protein (g)	Score
Cheeses						
Romano	1 oz	1	0	8	9	N
Swiss	1 oz	1	0	8	8	N
Ricotta, part skim milk	1 oz	1.5	0	2	3	N

Dairy Origin

	Serving Size	Usable Carbs (g)	Fiber (g)	Fat (g)	Protein (g)	Score
Butter	1 tbsp	0	0	12	0	F+
Heavy Whipping Cream	1 tbsp	0	0	6	0	F+
Sour Cream	2 tbsp	1	0	5	1	F+
Hood®						
Carb Countdown™, chocolate	1 cup	2	1	4.5	12	P
Cottage Cheese	1/2 cup	3	0	5	13	P
Cottage Cheese, low-fat	1/2 cup	3	0	1	14	P+
Dannon®						
Carb Control™ Yogurt (all flavors)	4 oz	3	0	3	5	N
Hood						
Carb Countdown, 2%	1 cup	3	0	4.5	12	P
Carb Countdown, skim	1 cup	3	0	0	12	P+

	Serving Size	Usable Carbs (g)	Fiber (g)	Fat (g)	Protein (g)	Score

Dairy Origin

	Serving Size	Usable Carbs (g)	Fiber (g)	Fat (g)	Protein (g)	Score
Carb Countdown Smoothies	1 bottle	4	0	3	14	P
Carb Countdown Yogurt	1 serving	4	0	1.5	12	P+

Egg Products

Egg Whites, chicken	1 large	0	0	0	4	P+
Egg, quail	1	0	0	1	1	N
Liquid Egg Substitutes	1 fl oz	0	0	2	6	P
Egg, fried or scrambled	1	0.5	0	7	6	F
Egg, hardboiled or poached	1	0.5	0	5	6	N
Egg Yolk, chicken	1 large	0.5	0	4.5	3	F
Egg, duck	1	1	0	10	9	F

Seafood

Alligator	3 oz	0	0	2	28	P+
Anchovy, canned in oil	3 oz	0	0	9	25	P
Anchovy, fresh	3 oz	0	0	4	17	P
Bass	3 oz	0	0	3	20	P
Bluefin	3 oz	0	0	5	25	P

Seafood

	Serving Size	Usable Carbs (g)	Fiber (g)	Fat (g)	Protein (g)	Score
Bluefish	3 oz	0	0	5	22	P
Butterfish	3 oz	0	0	9	19	N
Carp	3 oz	0	0	6	19	P
Catfish, farmed	3 oz	0	0	7	16	P
Catfish, wild	3 oz	0	0	3	16	P
Cod	3 oz	0	0	1	19	P+
Crab	3 oz	0	0	1	16	P+
Dolphin Fish	3 oz	0	0	1	20	P+
Flounder	3 oz	0	0	1	20	P+
Grouper	3 oz	0	0	1	21	P+
Haddock	3 oz	0	0	1	20	P+
Halibut, Greenland	3 oz	0	0	15	16	N
Halibut, Pacific	3 oz	0	0	3	23	P+
Herring	3 oz	0	0	10	20	N
Mackerel	3 oz	0	0	15	20	N
Monkfish	3 oz	0	0	2	16	P+
Pike	3 oz	0	0	1	21	P+
Pollack	3 oz	0	0	1	21	P+
Pompano	3 oz	0	0	10	20	N
Salmon, Atlantic	3 oz	0	0	10	19	N
Salmon, lox	3 oz	0	0	4	15	P
Salmon, pink	3 oz	0	0	4	21	P

Seafood

	Serving Size	Usable Carbs (g)	Fiber (g)	Fat (g)	Protein (g)	Score
Salmon, smoked	3 oz	0	0	4	15	P
Salmon, Wild Alaskan	3 oz	0	0	9	23	P
Sardines, canned in oil	3 oz	0	0	10	21	N
Shrimp	3 oz	0	0	1	18	P+
Snapper	3 oz	0	0	2	22	P+
Sole	3 oz	0	0	1	20	P+
Sturgeon	3 oz	0	0	5	18	P
Swordfish	3 oz	0	0	4	22	P
Trout	3 oz	0	0	7	23	P
Tuna, light, canned in oil	3 oz	0	0	7	25	P
Tuna, light, canned in water	3 oz	0	0	1	22	P+
Tuna, white, canned in oil	3 oz	0	0	7	22	P
Tuna, white, canned in water	3 oz	0	0	3	24	P+
Whitefish	3 oz	0	0	6	21	P
Yellowtail	3 oz	0	0	6	25	P
Scallops	3 oz	2	0	1	14	P+
Squid	3 oz	3	0	1	13	P+

Poultry

	Serving Size	Usable Carbs (g)	Fiber (g)	Fat (g)	Protein (g)	Score
Chicken Breast, skinless	1/2	0	0	3	27	P+
Chicken Breast, with skin	1/2	0	0	8	29	P
Chicken Drumstick, skinless	1	0	0	3	12	P
Chicken Drumstick, with skin	1	0	0	6	14	P
Chicken Giblets, fried	3 oz	0	0	11	28	P
Chicken Thigh, skinless	1	0	0	6	14	P
Chicken Thigh, with skin	1	0	0	10	15	N
Chicken Wing, skinless	1	0	0	2	6	P
Chicken Wing, with skin	1	0	0	7	9	N
Chicken, dark meat, diced	3 oz	0	0	8	23	P
Chicken, white meat, diced	3 oz	0	0	4	26	P
Cornish Hen, skinless	1 bird	0	0	9	50	P
Cornish Hen, with skin	1 bird	0	0	47	57	N

	Serving Size	Usable Carbs (g)	Fiber (g)	Fat (g)	Protein (g)	Score
Poultry						
Duck	3 oz	0	0	9	20	P
Ostrich	3 oz	0	0	3	24	P+
Pheasant, skinless	1/2 bird	0	0	13	83	P
Turkey, dark meat, diced	3 oz	0	0	6	24	P
Turkey, white meat	3 oz	0	0	3	25	P+
Turkey salami	3 oz	0	0	8	13	N
Hormel®						
Turkey Pepperoni	1 oz	0	0	4	9	P

Red Meat						
Beef, bottom round	3 oz	0	0	8	23	P
Beef, brisket	3 oz	0	0	8	27	P
Beef, filet mignon	3 oz	0	0	20	21	N
Beef, flank steak	3 oz	0	0	8	23	P
Beef, ground, 70% lean	3 oz	0	0	15	22	N
Beef, ground, 80% lean	3 oz	0	0	14	23	N
Beef, ground, 90% lean	3 oz	0	0	10	24	P

Red Meat

	Serving Size	Usable Carbs (g)	Fiber (g)	Fat (g)	Protein (g)	Score
Beef, ground, 95% lean	3 oz	0	0	6	25	P
Beef, patties	3 oz	0	0	16	20	N
Beef, porterhouse	3 oz	0	0	17	20	N
Beef, rib eye	3 oz	0	0	24	20	F
Beef, t-bone	3 oz	0	0	13	20	N
Beef, tri-tip	3 oz	0	0	9	22	P
Beefalo	3 oz	0	0	5	26	P
Buffalo	3 oz	0	0	5	24	P
Corned Beef	3 oz	0	0	16	15	N
Elk	3 oz	0	0	2	26	P+
Lamb	3 oz	0	0	14	21	N
Pastrami	3 oz	0	0	5	18	P
Rabbit	3 oz	0	0	7	25	P
Roast Beef, sliced 95% fat free	3 oz	0	0	4.5	13.5	P
Venison	3 oz	0	0	2	26	P+
Salami, beef	3 oz	2	0	19	11	F

Pork and Sausages

	Serving Size	Usable Carbs (g)	Fiber (g)	Fat (g)	Protein (g)	Score
Bacon	3 slices	0	0	10	9	F
Bacon Bits	1 tbsp	0	0	1.5	3	N
Boar	3 oz	0	0	4	24	P
Canadian Bacon	3 oz	0	0	7	21	P

Pork and Sausages

	Serving Size	Usable Carbs (g)	Fiber (g)	Fat (g)	Protein (g)	Score
Coppa	1 oz	0	0	6	8	N
Ham, extra lean (5% fat)	3 oz	0	0	5	18	P
Ham, regular (11% fat)	3 oz	0	0	8	19	P
Pepperoni	1 oz	0	0	13	5	F+
Pork Chops	3 oz	0	0	6	23	P
Pork Rinds	1 serving	0	0	4.5	9	N
Pork Sausage	1 link	0	0	7	5	F
Pork Tenderloins	3 oz	0	0	5	24	P
Oscar Mayer®						
Ready Serve Bacon	3 slices	0	0	5	5	N
Panceta	1 oz	1	0	13	4	F+
Prosciutto	1 oz	1	0	5	8	N
Salami, hard	1 oz	0.5	0	9.5	6	F
Salami, Italian	1 oz	0.5	0	10	6	F
Hormel						
Spam® Lite	3 oz	1	0	12	13	N
Chef Bruce Aidells® Sausages						
Artichoke & Garlic	1 link	1	2	9	14	N
Cajun Style	1 link	1	0	16	14	F

	Serving Size	Usable Carbs (g)	Fiber (g)	Fat (g)	Protein (g)	Score
Pork and Sausages						
Chicken & Apple	1 link	1	0	14	14	N
Sundried Tomato	1 link	1	0	13	17	N
Habanero & Green Chili	1 link	2	0	10	15	N
Pesto	1 link	2	0	13	16	N
Portobello Mushroom	1 link	2	1	8	14	N
Roasted Red Pepper	1 link	2	0	3.5	16	P
Hormel						
Spam	3 oz	3	0	23	11	F

Spices, Seasonings						
Basil, fresh	5 leaves	0	0	0	0	N
Bay Leaves	1 tsp	0	0	0	0	N
Black Pepper	1 tsp	0	0	0	0	N
Capers	1 tbsp	0	0	0	0	N
Cayenne	1 tsp	0	0	0	0	N
Celery Salt	1 tsp	0	0	0	0	N
Cilantro	1 tsp	0	0	0	0	N
Curry Powder, yellow	1 tsp	0	0	0	0	N

	Serving Size	Usable Carbs (g)	Fiber (g)	Fat (g)	Protein (g)	Score

Spices, Seasonings

	Serving Size	Usable Carbs (g)	Fiber (g)	Fat (g)	Protein (g)	Score
Dill	1 tsp	0	0	0	0	N
Fennel	1 tsp	0	0	0	0	N
Garlic Salt	1 tsp	0	0	0	0	N
Japanese Wasabi	1 tsp	0	0	0	0	N
Nutmeg	1 tsp	0	0	0	0	N
Onion Salt	1 tsp	0	0	0	0	N
Oregano	1 tsp	0	0	0	0	N
Paprika	1 tsp	0	0	0	0	N
Parsley	1 tsp	0	0	0	0	N
Peppermint, fresh	5 leaves	0	0	0	0	N
Red Pepper	1 tsp	0	0	0	0	N
Rosemary	1 tsp	0	0	0	0	N
Salt	1 tsp	0	0	0	0	N
Spearmint, fresh	5 leaves	0	0	0	0	N
Wasabi Powder	1 tsp	0	0	0	0	N
White Pepper	1 tsp	0	0	0	0	N
Chef Paul PrudHomme's®						
Magic Seasoning Blends	1 tsp	0	0	0	0	N
Gringo Billy's™						
Low Carb Taco Seasoning	1 tsp	0	1	0	0	N

Baking Goods

	Serving Size	Usable Carbs (g)	Fiber (g)	Fat (g)	Protein (g)	Score
Baking Soda	1 tsp	0	0	0	0	N
Flaxseed Meal	2 tbsp	0	4	4.5	3	F
Guar Gum	1 tbsp	0	6	0	0	N
Xanthan Gum	1 tsp	0	3	0	0	N
Let's Go...Organic™						
Lite Coconut, shredded	2.5 tbsp	0	0	6	1	F+
Pure Vanilla Extract	1 tsp	0.5	0	0	0	N
Baking Powder	1 tsp	1	0	0	0	N
Cocoa Powder, unsweetened	1 tbsp	1	2	1	1	N
Instant Coffee, powder	1 tsp	1	0	0	0	N
Coconut, unsweetened, shredded	1 oz	2	5	18	2	F+
Bob's Red Mill®						
Coconut, unsweetened	1/4 cup	2	2	11	1	F+
Almond meal	1/4 cup	2	3	15	7	F
Hazelnut meal	1/4 cup	2	3	18	4	F+
Granulated Splenda® (for baking)	1/4 cup	6	0	0	0	N

	Serving Size	Usable Carbs (g)	Fiber (g)	Fat (g)	Protein (g)	Score
Beverages						
Coffee, decaffeinated	8 fl oz	0	0	0	0	N
Club Soda	8 fl oz	0	0	0	0	N
Diet Tonic Water	8 fl oz	0	0	0	0	N
Herbal Green Tea	8 fl oz	0	0	0	0	N
Atkins®						
Sugar Free Lemon Iced Tea	8 fl oz	0	0	0	0	N
Carb Options™						
Lemon Iced Tea	8 fl oz	0	0	0	0	N
Celestial Seasons®						
Herbal Teas	8 fl oz	0	0	0	0	N
Hansen's®						
Diet Sodas, all flavors	1 can	0	0	0	0	N
Snapple® Diet Iced Teas						
Lemon	8 fl oz	0	0	0	0	N
Lime Green Tea	8 fl oz	0	0	0	0	N
Peach	8 fl oz	0	0	0	0	N
Plum-A-Granate	8 fl oz	0	0	0	0	N
Raspberry	8 fl oz	0	0	0	0	N

	Serving Size	Usable Carbs (g)	Fiber (g)	Fat (g)	Protein (g)	Score
Treats						
Sugar Free Jello®	1 serving	0	0	0	1	P+
Strawberries	1/2 cup	4	1	0	0	N

Condiments

	Serving Size	Usable Carbs (g)	Fiber (g)	Fat (g)	Protein (g)	Score
Atkins						
BBQ Sauce	1 tbsp	0	0	0	0	N
Carb Options						
Asian Teriyaki Marinade	1 tbsp	0	0	0	0	N
Italian Garlic Marinade	1 tbsp	0	0	0	0	N
Carb Well™						
A1® Steak Sauce	1 tbsp	0	0	0	0	N
Hellman's®						
Mayonnaise	1 tbsp	0	0	11	0	F+
Hot Sauce, most	1 tbsp	0	0	0	0	N
Mustard, most	1 tbsp	0	0	0	0	N
Red Wine Vinegar	1 tbsp	0	0	0	0	N
Rice Vinegar, unflavored	1 tbsp	0	0	0	0	N
Saffola®						
Mayonnaise	1 tbsp	0	0	11	0	F+
Walden Farms®						
Ketchup	1 tbsp	0	0	0	0	N
Seafood Sauce	1 tbsp	0	0	0	0	N

	Serving Size	Usable Carbs (g)	Fiber (g)	Fat (g)	Protein (g)	Score
Condiments						
White Wine Vinegar	1 tbsp	0	0	0	0	N
Soy Sauce, regular	1 tbsp	1	0	0	1	P+
Lemon Juice	1 tbsp	2	0	0	0	N
Lime Juice	1 tbsp	2	0	0	0	N
Au Jus	1/2 cup	3	0	0	1	P+

Salad Dressings

	Serving Size	Usable Carbs (g)	Fiber (g)	Fat (g)	Protein (g)	Score
Carb Options						
Italian	2 tbsp	0	0	8	0	F+
Olive Oil Vinaigrette	2 tbsp	0	0	6	0	F+
Ranch	2 tbsp	0	0	17	0	F+
Carb Well						
Ceasar	2 tbsp	0	0	11	0	F+
Creamy French	2 tbsp	0	0	11	0	F+
Italian	2 tbsp	0	0	8	0	F+
Italian Lite	2 tbsp	0	0	1.5	0	F+
Ranch	2 tbsp	0	0	11	0	F+

	Serving Size	Usable Carbs (g)	Fiber (g)	Fat (g)	Protein (g)	Score

Pasta and Pizza Sauces

	Serving Size	Usable Carbs (g)	Fiber (g)	Fat (g)	Protein (g)	Score
Carb Options / Ragu®						
Alfredo Sauce	1/4 cup	2	0	10	1	F+
Rao's®						
Homemade Arrabbiata	1/2 cup	3	1	4.5	1	F+
Alessi®						
Puttanesca	1/2 cup	4	2	9	2	F+
Middle Earth Organics™						
Porcini Mushroom	1/2 cup	4	1	4	1	F+
Tomato & Basil	1/2 cup	4	1	4	1	F+
Tomato & Eggplant	1/2 cup	4	1	4	1	F+
Rao's						
Homemade Puttanesca	1/2 cup	4	1	4.5	2	F+
Silver Palate™						
Balsamico	1/2 cup	4	1	4	1	F+
Carb Options / Ragu						
Italian Style Pizza Sauce with Sausage	1/2 cup	5	2	13	5	F+

	Serving Size	Usable Carbs (g)	Fiber (g)	Fat (g)	Protein (g)	Score

Pasta and Pizza Sauces

	Serving Size	Usable Carbs (g)	Fiber (g)	Fat (g)	Protein (g)	Score
Francis Coppola®						
Arrabbiata	1/2 cup	5	1	2.5	1	F+
Pomadora-Basilico	1/2 cup	5	0	2.5	1	F+
Puttanesca	1/2 cup	5	1	2.5	1	F+
Patsy's®						
Tomato & Basil	1/2 cup	5	2	6	2	F+

Syrups

	Serving Size	Usable Carbs (g)	Fiber (g)	Fat (g)	Protein (g)	Score
Atkins						
Sugar-Free Pancake Syrup	1/4 cup	0	0	0	0	N
Da Vinci®						
Sugar Free Syrups	1 oz	0	0	0	0	N
Ketogenics						
Pancake Syrup	1/4 cup	0	0	0	0	N
Torani®						
Sugar Free Syrups	1 oz	0	0	0	0	N

Oils

Choosing the right oils is important for health. The oils are ordered according to the concentration of omega-3 fats.

- The serving size for all oils is one tablespoon
- Try to use oils higher on the list when possible.
- For high temperature cooking, like frying, use only avocado, hazelnut, safflower and olive oils; other oils can break down into large amounts of trans-fat.
- Do not use flaxseed oil for cooking
- Refrigerate oils and discard after three months

	Total Fat (g)	Saturated (g)	Mono-unsaturated (g)	Omega-3 (g)	Omega-6 (g)	Score
Flaxseed	13.6	1.3	2.7	7.2	1.7	F+
Canola	13.6	1	8	1.3	2.7	F+
Pumpkin Seed	13.6	1.2	4.6	2.2	5.8	F+
Hemp	13.6	1.1	1.6	2.7	8.2	F+
Walnut	13.6	1.2	3.1	1.4	7.2	F+
Soybean	13.6	2	3.2	0.9	6.9	F+
Olive	13.6	1.8	10	0.1	1.2	F+
Avocado	13.6	1.6	9.6	0.1	1.7	F+
Teaseed	13.6	2.9	7	0.1	3	F+
Grapeseed	13.6	1.3	2.2	0	9.5	F+
Sunflower	13.6	1.4	2.7	0	8.9	F+
Sesame	13.6	1.9	5.4	0	5.6	F+
Peanut	13.6	2.3	6.2	0	4.3	F+
Almond	13.6	1.1	9.5	0	2.4	F+
Safflower	13.6	0.8	10.2	0	1.9	F+
Hazelnut	13.6	1	10.6	0	1.4	F+
Cocoa Butter	13.6	8.1	4.5	0	0.4	F+

Ultralow-Carb Protein Powders

- Serving size is 1 scoop

	Flavors	Usable Carbs (g)	Fiber (g)	Fat (g)	Protein (g)	Score
Isopure®						
from Nature's Best®	Alpine Punch	0	0	0.5	25	P+
	Apple Melon	0	0	0.5	25	P+
Ordering Information:	Creamy Vanilla	0	0	0	25	P+
www.naturesbest.com	Mango Peach	0	0	0.5	25	P+
	Pineapple Orange Banana	0	0	0.5	25	P+
	Strawberries & Cream	0	0	0	25	P+
	Dutch Chocolate	0.5	1	0	25	P+
Nectar™						
from Syntrax	Apple Ecstasy	0	0	0	23	P+
	Caribbean Cooler	0	0	0	23	P+
Ordering Information:	Crystal Sky Fruit Punch	0	0	0	23	P+
www.syntrax.com	Fuzzy Navel	0	0	0	23	P+
	Roadside Lemonade	0	0	0	23	P+
	Strawberry Kiwi	0	0	0	23	P+
	Very Cherry Berry	0	0	0	23	P+
Pure WPI						
from Bioplex Nutrition™	Chocolate	0	0	0	20	P+
	Natural	0	0	0	20	P+
Ordering Information:	Vanilla	0	0	0	20	P+
www.bioplexnutrition.com	Very Berry	0	0	0	20	P+

PM Protein™

	Flavors	Usable Carbs (g)	Fiber (g)	Fat (g)	Protein (g)	Score
from GNC®	Vanilla Caramel	0.5	0.5	1	20	P+
	Strawberry	0.5	0.5	1	20	P+
Ordering Information:						
www.gnc.com						

Ultralow-Carb Caffeinated Drinks

	Serving size	Usable Carbs (g)	Fiber (g)	Fat (g)	Protein (g)	Caffeine (mg)
Coffee, Drip	8 fl oz	0	0	0	0	95
Coffee, Espresso	2 fl oz	0	0	0	0	127

The Source Drinks®

Burn®	1 can	0	0	0	1	118

Ordering Information:

   www.sourcedrinks.com

Stacker 2®

YJ Stinger™ Sugar Free	1 can	0	0	0	0	100

Ordering Information:

   www.yjstinger.com

ABB®

Diet Turbo Tea™	1 bottle	0	0	0	0	90
Speedstack™	1 bottle	1	0	0	0	250
Extreme Speedstack™	1 bottle	2	0	0	0	300

Ordering Information:

   www.americanbodybuilding.com

	Serving size	Usable Carbs (g)	Fiber (g)	Fat (g)	Protein (g)	Caffeine (mg)
Sobe®						
Adrenaline Rush™, Sugar Free	1 can	1	0	0	0	79
No Fear®, Sugar Free	1 can	2	0	0	2	158

Ordering Information:

www.sobebev.com

Red Bull®

	Serving size	Usable Carbs (g)	Fiber (g)	Fat (g)	Protein (g)	Caffeine (mg)
Sugar Free	1 can	3	0	0	0	80

Ordering Information:

www.redbullusa.com

Monster Energy™

	Serving size	Usable Carbs (g)	Fiber (g)	Fat (g)	Protein (g)	Caffeine (mg)
Lo-Carb	1 can	3	0	0	0	120

Ordering Information:

www.monsterenergy.com

Fiber Supplements

	Serving size	Usable Carbs (g)	Fiber (g)	Fat (g)	Protein (g)
Colon Cleanse®					
Psyllium Husk	1 tbsp	0	6	0	0

Ordering Information:

www.gnc.com

Konsyl®					
Psyllium Husk	1 tsp	0	5	0	0

Ordering Information:

www.konsyl.com

Benefiber®					
Hydrolyzed Guar Gum	1 tbsp	1	3	0	0

Information:

www.benefiber.com

Metamucil®					
Psyllium Husk	1 tsp	2	3	0	0

Information:

www.metamucil.com

Breath Aids

	Serving size	Usable Carbs (g)	Fiber (g)	Fat (g)	Protein (g)

Ice Breakers®

	Serving size	Usable Carbs (g)	Fiber (g)	Fat (g)	Protein (g)
Liquid Ice Mints	1 mint	0	0	0	0

Information:

www.hersheys.com

Breath Asure®

	Serving size	Usable Carbs (g)	Fiber (g)	Fat (g)	Protein (g)
MintAsure™	3 mints	0	0	0	0

Ordering Information:

www.breathasure.com

Carb Nite Fruit Guide

On a Carb Nite: Try to select fruits toward the top of the list and eat those toward the bottom of the list sparingly. Remember to always avoid fruit on fat and protein days.

- All values are for a 100 gram portion.
- Fruits with a larger ratio of glucose to fructose are healthier on any diet.

	Fiber (g)	Glucose (g)	Fructose (g)	Sucrose (g)	Ratio (x100)
Plums	1	5	3	2	152
Apricots	2	2	1	6	137
Cherries	2	7	5	0	122
Peach	2	2	2	5	111
Figs, dried	10	25	23	0	108
Nectarine	2	2	1	5	105
Banana	3	5	5	2	102
Dates	8	20	20	24	101
Blueberries	2	5	5	0	98
Tangerine	2	2	2	6	95
Kiwi	3	4	4	0	95
Orange	2	2	2	4	94
Raisins	4	28	30	0	94
Pineapple	1	2	2	5	94
Cantaloupe	1	2	2	4	92
Grapes	1	7	8	0	89
Strawberries	2	2	3	0	82
Raspberries	7	2	2	0	80
Watermelon	0	2	3	1	55
Apple	2	2	6	2	49
Pear	3	3	6	1	48

Food Score Calculator

To determine the food score of items not found on the included food list, use the Food Score Calculator on the following pages.

How it works

On the nutrition label, find the total grams of fat and protein. Along the top of row of the Calculator, find the column with the corresponding number of grams of protein. On the right hand side, find the row of the corresponding number of grams of fat. Trace down the appropriate column and over in the appropriate row until the two meet—this is the score for the particular item.

Grams of Protein Per Serving

16	15	14	13	12	11	10	9	8	7	6	5	4	3	2	1	0	
P+	P+	P+	P+	P+	P+	P+	P+	P+	P+	P+	P+	P+	P+	P+	P+	N	0
P+	P+	P+	P+	P+	P+	P+	P+	P+	P	P	P	P	P	N	N	F	1
P+	P+	P	P	P	P	P	P	P	P	P	P	N	N	N	F	F+	2
P	P	P	P	P	P	P	P	P	P	N	N	N	N	F	F+	F+	3
P	P	P	P	P	P	P	P	N	N	N	N	N	F	F	F+	F+	4
P	P	P	P	P	P	N	N	N	N	N	N	F	F	F+	F+	F+	5
P	P	P	P	N	N	N	N	N	N	N	F	F	F	F+	F+	F+	6
P	P	N	N	N	N	N	N	N	N	F	F	F	F+	F+	F+	F+	7
N	N	N	N	N	N	N	N	N	F	F	F	F	F+	F+	F+	F+	8

Grams of Fat Per Serving

Finding the Food Score For a Product with 5 grams of fat and 13 grams of protein

Grams of Fat Per Serving

Grams of Protein Per Serving

P\F	0	1	2	3	4	5	6	7	8	9	10	11	12	13	14	15	16	17	18	19	20	21	22	23
0	N	F+	F+	F+	F+	F+	F+	F+	F+	F+	F+	F+	F+	F+	F+	F+	F+	F+	F+	F+	F+	F+	F+	F+
1	P+	N	F	F+	F+	F+	F+	F+	F+	F+	F+	F+	F+	F+	F+	F+	F+	F+	F+	F+	F+	F+	F+	F+
2	P+	Z	Z	F	F	F+	F+	F+	F+	F+	F+	F+	F+	F+	F+	F+	F+	F+	F+	F+	F+	F+	F+	F+
3	P+	P	Z	Z	Z	F	F	F	F+	F+	F+	F+	F+	F+	F+	F+	F+	F+	F+	F+	F+	F+	F+	F+
4	P+	P	Z	Z	Z	Z	F	F	F	F	F+	F+	F+	F+	F+	F+	F+	F+	F+	F+	F+	F+	F+	F+
5	P+	P	P	Z	Z	Z	Z	F	F	F	F	F	F+	F+	F+	F+	F+	F+	F+	F+	F+	F+	F+	F+
6	P+	P	P	Z	Z	Z	Z	Z	F	F	F	F	F	F	F+	F+	F+	F+	F+	F+	F+	F+	F+	F+
7	P+	P	P	P	Z	Z	Z	Z	Z	F	F	F	F	F	F	F+	F+	F+	F+	F+	F+	F+	F+	F+
8	P+	P+	P	P	Z	Z	Z	Z	Z	Z	F	F	F	F	F	F	F	F+	F+	F+	F+	F+	F+	F+
9	P+	P+	P	P	P	Z	Z	Z	Z	Z	Z	F	F	F	F	F	F	F	F	F+	F+	F+	F+	F+
10	P+	P+	P	P	P	P	Z	Z	Z	Z	Z	Z	F	F	F	F	F	F	F	F	F	F	F	F
11	P+	P+	P	P	P	P	Z	Z	Z	Z	Z	Z	Z	F	F	F	F	F	F	F	F	F	F	F
12	P+	P+	P	P	P	P	Z	Z	Z	Z	Z	Z	Z	Z	F	F	F	F	F	F	F	F	F	F
13	P+	P+	P	P	P	P	P	Z	Z	Z	Z	Z	Z	Z	Z	F	F	F	F	F	F	F	F	F
14	P+	P+	P	P	P	P	P	Z	Z	Z	Z	Z	Z	Z	Z	Z	F	F	F	F	F	F	F	F
15	P+	P+	P+	P	P	P	P	P	Z	Z	Z	Z	Z	Z	Z	Z	Z	F	F	F	F	F	F	F
16	P+	P+	P+	P	P	P	P	P	Z	Z	Z	Z	Z	Z	Z	Z	Z	Z	F	F	F	F	F	F
17	P+	P+	P+	P	P	P	P	P	Z	Z	Z	Z	Z	Z	Z	Z	Z	Z	Z	F	F	F	F	F
18	P+	P+	P+	P	P	P	P	P	P	Z	Z	Z	Z	Z	Z	Z	Z	Z	Z	Z	F	F	F	F
19	P+	P+	P+	P	P	P	P	P	P	Z	Z	Z	Z	Z	Z	Z	Z	Z	Z	Z	Z	F	F	F
20	P+	P+	P+	P	P	P	P	P	P	P	Z	Z	Z	Z	Z	Z	Z	Z	Z	Z	Z	Z	F	F
21	P+	P+	P+	P	P	P	P	P	P	P	Z	Z	Z	Z	Z	Z	Z	Z	Z	Z	Z	Z	Z	F
22	P+	P+	P+	P	P	P	P	P	P	P	P	Z	Z	Z	Z	Z	Z	Z	Z	Z	Z	Z	Z	Z
23	P+	P+	P+	P+	P	P	P	P	P	P	P	P	Z	Z	Z	Z	Z	Z	Z	Z	Z	Z	Z	Z
24	P+	P+	P+	P+	P	P	P	P	P	P	P	P	Z	Z	Z	Z	Z	Z	Z	Z	Z	Z	Z	Z
25	P+	P+	P+	P+	P	P	P	P	P	P	P	P	Z	Z	Z	Z	Z	Z	Z	Z	Z	Z	Z	Z
26	P+	P+	P+	P+	P	P	P	P	P	P	P	P	P	Z	Z	Z	Z	Z	Z	Z	Z	Z	Z	Z
27	P+	P+	P+	P+	P	P	P	P	P	P	P	P	P	Z	Z	Z	Z	Z	Z	Z	Z	Z	Z	Z
28	P+	P+	P+	P+	P	P	P	P	P	P	P	P	P	P	Z	Z	Z	Z	Z	Z	Z	Z	Z	Z
29	P+	P+	P+	P+	P	P	P	P	P	P	P	P	P	P	Z	Z	Z	Z	Z	Z	Z	Z	Z	Z
30	P+	P+	P+	P+	P+	P	P	P	P	P	P	P	P	P	P	Z	Z	Z	Z	Z	Z	Z	Z	Z

Keep in Book

Food Score Calculator

Grams of Fat Per Serving

Row labels (left) = Grams of Protein Per Serving (0–30). Columns = Grams of Fat Per Serving (0–23). Cell values: N, F, F+, P, P+.

Protein \ Fat	0	1	2	3	4	5	6	7	8	9	10	11	12	13	14	15	16	17	18	19	20	21	22	23
0	N	F+	F+	F+	F+	F+	F+	F+	F+	F+	F+	F+	F+	F+	F+	F+	F+	F+	F+	F+	F+	F+	F+	F+
1	P+	N	F	F+	F+	F+	F+	F+	F+	F+	F+	F+	F+	F+	F+	F+	F+	F+	F+	F+	F+	F+	F+	F+
2	P+	N	N	F	F+	F+	F+	F+	F+	F+	F+	F+	F+	F+	F+	F+	F+	F+	F+	F+	F+	F+	F+	F+
3	P+	P	N	N	F	F	F	F+	F+	F+	F+	F+	F+	F+	F+	F+	F+	F+	F+	F+	F+	F+	F+	F+
4	P+	P	N	N	N	F	F	F	F	F+	F+	F+	F+	F+	F+	F+	F+	F+	F+	F+	F+	F+	F+	F+
5	P+	P	P	N	N	N	N	F	F	F	F	F+	F+	F+	F+	F+	F+	F+	F+	F+	F+	F+	F+	F+
6	P+	P	P	N	N	N	N	F	F	F	F	F	F	F+	F+	F+	F+	F+	F+	F+	F+	F+	F+	F+
7	P+	P	P	P	N	N	N	N	F	F	F	F	F	F	F	F+	F+	F+	F+	F+	F+	F+	F+	F+
8	P+	P+	P	P	N	N	N	N	N	F	F	F	F	F	F	F	F	F+	F+	F+	F+	F+	F+	F+
9	P+	P+	P	P	P	N	N	N	N	N	F	F	F	F	F	F	F	F	F	F+	F+	F+	F+	F+
10	P+	P+	P	P	P	N	N	N	N	N	N	F	F	F	F	F	F	F	F	F	F	F+	F+	F+
11	P+	P+	P	P	P	P	N	N	N	N	N	N	N	F	F	F	F	F	F	F	F	F	F	F
12	P+	P+	P	P	P	P	N	N	N	N	N	N	N	N	F	F	F	F	F	F	F	F	F	F
13	P+	P+	P	P	P	P	P	N	N	N	N	N	N	N	N	F	F	F	F	F	F	F	F	F
14	P+	P+	P	P	P	P	P	N	N	N	N	N	N	N	N	N	F	F	F	F	F	F	F	F
15	P+	P+	P+	P	P	P	P	P	N	N	N	N	N	N	N	N	N	F	F	F	F	F	F	F
16	P+	P+	P+	P	P	P	P	P	N	N	N	N	N	N	N	N	N	N	F	F	F	F	F	F
17	P+	P+	P+	P	P	P	P	P	N	N	N	N	N	N	N	N	N	N	F	F	F	F	F	F
18	P+	P+	P+	P	P	P	P	P	P	N	N	N	N	N	N	N	N	N	N	F	F	F	F	F
19	P+	P+	P+	P	P	P	P	P	P	N	N	N	N	N	N	N	N	N	N	F	F	F	F	F
20	P+	P+	P+	P	P	P	P	P	P	P	N	N	N	N	N	N	N	N	N	N	N	F	F	F
21	P+	P+	P+	P	P	P	P	P	P	P	N	N	N	N	N	N	N	N	N	N	N	N	F	F
22	P+	P+	P+	P	P	P	P	P	P	P	P	N	N	N	N	N	N	N	N	N	N	N	N	N
23	P+	P+	P+	P+	P	P	P	P	P	P	P	N	N	N	N	N	N	N	N	N	N	N	N	N
24	P+	P+	P+	P+	P	P	P	P	P	P	P	N	N	N	N	N	N	N	N	N	N	N	N	N
25	P+	P+	P+	P+	P	P	P	P	P	P	P	P	N	N	N	N	N	N	N	N	N	N	N	N
26	P+	P+	P+	P+	P	P	P	P	P	P	P	P	N	N	N	N	N	N	N	N	N	N	N	N
27	P+	P+	P+	P+	P	P	P	P	P	P	P	P	N	N	N	N	N	N	N	N	N	N	N	N
28	P+	P+	P+	P+	P	P	P	P	P	P	P	P	P	N	N	N	N	N	N	N	N	N	N	N
29	P+	P+	P+	P+	P	P	P	P	P	P	P	P	P	N	N	N	N	N	N	N	N	N	N	N
30	P+	P+	P+	P+	P	P	P	P	P	P	P	P	P	P	N	N	N	N	N	N	N	N	N	N

Cut Out For Use When Shopping

Food Score Calculator

Meal Plans

Simple Menu Plans, Lower Calorie

- Quick and easy preparation
- Convenient for traveling
- Fewer daily meals
- Ideal for busy lifestyles
- Appropriate for 150 lb persons and below

Items in *italics* can be found in the Recipes section.

Simple Menu Planning, Lower Calorie

Day 1

Breakfast

1 serving	*Goat Cheese & Spinach Omelette* page 236
1 cup	Carb Countdown Skim Milk
1 serving	Colon Cleanse Psyllium Fiber

Lunch

1 serving	*Ceasar Tuna Pouch Shaker* page 302
2 oz	Jarlsberg Cheese (1 slice)
1 can	Hansen's Diet Soda

Dinner

1	Chicken Breast
2 oz	Shredded cheddar cheese
1 tbsp	Hot Sauce
1 serving	Benefiber

Bedtime

1 bottle	Carb Countdown Fruit Smoothie
1 serving	Benefiber

	Usable Carbs	Fiber	Fat	Protein
Totals for the day (in grams)	10	12	99	144

Simple Menu Planning, Lower Calorie

Day 2

Breakfast

6 slices	Oscar Mayer Ready Serve Bacon
1 serving	*Golden Scrambled Eggs* page 238
1 cup	Carb Countdown Chocolate Milk
1 serving	Colon Cleanse Psyllium Fiber

Lunch

3 oz	Beef Salami
20 nuts	Pistachios

Dinner

½ lb	Hamburger patty (95% lean)
2 slices	Swiss cheese
	Mustard to taste
1 bottle	Snapple Diet Iced Tea
1 serving	Benefiber

Bedtime

1 serving	*Hazelnut Iced Cream* page 338

	Usable Carbs	Fiber	Fat	Protein
Totals for the day (in grams)	9	11	100	148

Simple Menu Planning, Lower Calorie

Day 3

Breakfast

6 oz	Ham Steak
1 oz	Colby Cheese
2	Hard-boiled eggs

Lunch

2 links	Chef Bruce Aidells Habanero & Green Chili Sausage
1 oz	Cheddar Cheese
	Mustard to taste

Dinner

1	*Mini-Alfredo Pepperoni & Basil Pizza* page 290
1 scoop	Nectar Roadside Lemonade

Bedtime

1 serving	*Fruitless Fiber Smoothie* page 344

	Usable Carbs	Fiber	Fat	Protein
Totals for the day (in grams)	13	14	99	150

Simple Menu Planning, Lower Calorie

Day 4

Breakfast

6 oz	Ham Steak
1 serving	*Fat Irish Coffee* page 342

Lunch

1 serving	*Salmon Teryaki Shaker* page 300
16 nuts	Macadamia

Dinner

4 servings	*Dijon Chicken Spinach Salad* page 258
1 serving	Sugar Free Jello

	Usable Carbs	Fiber	Fat	Protein
Totals for the day (in grams)	3	12	98	144

Simple Menu Planning, Lower Calorie

Day 5

Breakfast

2 servings	*Western Breakfast Wraps* page 250

Lunch

2 oz	Hormel Turkey Pepperoni
1 oz	Provolone Cheese

Dinner

5 oz	Turkey
2 oz	Colby Cheese
1 serving	Sugar Free Jello

Bedtime

1 scoop	GNC PM Protein
35 nuts	Almonds

	Usable Carbs	Fiber	Fat	Protein
Totals for the day (in grams)	11	17	98	143

Simple Menu Planning, Lower Calorie

Day 6

Breakfast

4	Fried Eggs
3 oz	Canadian Bacon

Lunch

5 servings	*Spicy Asian Lettuce Wraps* page 310

Dinner

2	*Chicken Fajitas* page 282

Bedtime

1 oz	Monterey Jack Cheese
1 bottle	Snapple Diet Iced Tea

	Usable Carbs	Fiber	Fat	Protein
Totals for the day (in grams)	14	19	96	150

Simple Menu Planning, Lower Calorie

Day 7

Breakfast

2 pancakes	*Ultralow-Carb Pancakes* page 242
1 cup	Carb Countdown 2% Milk
3 slices	Oscar Mayer Ready Serve Bacon
1 serving	Benefiber

Lunch

1 serving	*Ranch Tuna Pouch Shaker* page 302
1 tbsp	Real Bacon Bits

Dinner

2 links	Chef Bruce Aidells Habanero & Green Chili Sausage
	Mustard to taste
1 scoop	Nectar Protein
1 serving	Colon Cleanse Psyllium Fiber

Bedtime

1 cup	Carb Countdown Chocolate Milk, served warm

	Usable Carbs	Fiber	Fat	Protein
Totals for the day (in grams)	11	16	96	148

Simple Menu Planning, Lower Calorie

Day 8

Breakfast

4	Hard-boiled eggs
2 oz	Canadian Bacon
1 serving	Colon Cleanse Pysllium Fiber

Lunch

3 oz	Spam
2	Hard-boiled eggs
1 bottle	Carb Countdown Fruit Smoothie
1 serving	Benefiber

Dinner

1 serving	*Monte Cris-Lo* page 292

Bedtime

25 nuts	Almonds
1 cup	Cottage Cheese

	Usable Carbs	Fiber	Fat	Protein
Totals for the day (in grams)	14	12	96	147

Simple Menu Planning, Lower Calorie

Day 9

Breakfast

1 serving	*Pepper Cheddar Omelette* page 244
1 oz	Hard Salami
1 scoop	Nectar Protein Powder
1 serving	Colon Cleanse Pysillium Fiber

Lunch

4 servings	*Dijon Chicken Spinach Salad* page 258

Dinner

1 serving	*Bell Pepper Tacos* page 278

	Usable Carbs	Fiber	Fat	Protein
Totals for the day (in grams)	6	12	104	155

Simple Menu Planning, Lower Calorie

Day 10

Breakfast

6 oz	Ham Steak	
1 serving	*Hazelnut Iced Cream*	page 338

Lunch

3 wraps	*Spicy Asian Chicken Wraps*	page 310
10 nuts	Pecans	

Snack

1 bottle	Carb Countdown Fruit Smoothie

It's
Carb Nite!

Simple Menu Plans, Higher Calorie

- Quick and easy preparation
- Convenient for traveling
- Excellent hunger control
- Appropriate for 150+ lb individuals

Items in *italics* can be found in the Recipes section.

Simple Menu Planning, Higher Calorie

Day 1

Breakfast

4	Fried Eggs
3 oz	Canadian Bacon
1 serving	*Fat Irish Coffee* page 342

Snack

2 oz	Cheese stick
14 slices	*Pepperoni Chips* page 272

Lunch

½ lb	Hamburger patty (95% lean)
2 slices	Swiss cheese
	Mustard to taste
1 serving	Colon Cleanse Psyllium Fiber

Snack

¼ cup	Pumpkin Seeds
3 oz	Turkey

Dinner

1	*Crustless Pizza* page 284

	Usable Carbs	Fiber	Fat	Protein
Totals for the day (in grams)	6	12	130	208

Simple Menu Planning, Higher Calorie

Day 2

Breakfast

6 oz	Ham Steak
1 oz	Colby Cheese
2	Hard-boiled eggs

Snack

1 serving	*Fruity Cottage Cheese* page 270

Lunch

6 oz	Light Tuna in water
3 oz	Feta Cheese
1 cup	Carb Countdown Fruit Smoothie

Snack

2 oz	Hormel Turkey Pepperoni
1 oz	Provolone Cheese

Dinner

1	Chicken Breast
2 oz	Shredded cheddar cheese
1 tbsp	Hot Sauce
1 bottle	Snapple Diet Iced Tea
1 serving	Colon Cleanse Psyllium Fiber

Bedtime

2 servings	*Hazelnut Iced Cream* page 338

	Usable Carbs	Fiber	Fat	Protein
Totals for the day (in grams)	10	8	127	220

181

Simple Menu Planning, Higher Calorie

Day 3

Breakfast

1	*Goat Cheese & Spinach Omelette* page 236
1 cup	Carb Countdown Skim Milk

Snack

2 oz	Pepper Jack Cheese

Lunch

1 serving	*Monte Cris Lo* page 292
1 can	Hansen's Diet Soda

Snack

35 nuts	Almonds (about 1/3 of a cup)

Dinner

2	*Chicken Fajitas* page 282
1 scoop	Nectar Crystal Sky Fruit Punch

	Usable Carbs	Fiber	Fat	Protein
Totals for the day (in grams)	13	23	132	177

Simple Menu Planning, Higher Calorie

Day 4

Breakfast

3 oz	Spam
2	Hard-boiled eggs
1 cup	Cottage Cheese
1 bottle	Carb Countdown Fruit Smoothie
1 serving	Colon Cleanse Psyllium Fiber

Snack

3 oz	Turkey
1 oz	Colby Cheese
1 serving	Sugar Free Jello

Lunch

1 serving	*Ranch Tuna Pouch Shaker* page 302
1 bottle	Carb Countdown Yogurt

Snack

3 oz	Smoked Salmon
1 oz	Cream Cheese
1 serving	Benefiber

Dinner

1 serving	*Bell Pepper Tacos* page 278

Bedtime

2 serving	*Hazelnut Iced Cream* page 338
1 cup	Carb Countdown 2% Milk
1 serving	Colon Cleanse Psyllium Fiber

	Usable Carbs	Fiber	Fat	Protein
Totals for the day (in grams)	22	15	128	191

183

The Carb Nite Solution

Day 5

Breakfast

1 serving	*Golden Scrambled Eggs* page 238
6 slices	Oscar Mayer Ready Serve Bacon
1 cup	Carb Countdown Chocolate Milk
1 serving	Benefiber

Snack

2	Hard boiled eggs
1 can	Hansen's Diet Soda

Lunch

4 servings	*Dijon Chicken Spinach Salad* page 258

Snack

4 oz	Corned Beef
	Mustard to taste

Dinner

3 oz	Broiled Salmon
2 oz	Feta
1 serving	Colon Cleanse Psyllium Fiber

Bedtime

1 serving	*Hazelnut Iced Cream* page 338
1 scoop	Vanilla Caramel GNC PM Protein

	Usable Carbs	Fiber	Fat	Protein
Totals for the day (in grams)	6	13	132	189

184

Simple Menu Planning, Higher Calorie

Day 6

Breakfast

2 servings	*Western Breakfast Wraps* page 250
1 bottle	Carb Countdown Fruit Smoothie

Snack

14 slices	Hormel Turkey Pepperoni
1 oz	Mozzarella

Lunch

1 serving	*Ceasar Tuna Pouch Shaker* page 302

Snack

1 oz	Provolone Cheese

Dinner

2 links	Chef Bruce Aidells Artichoke & Garlic Sausage
20 nuts	Pecans
1 scoop	Nectar Protein

Bedtime

1 serving	*Hazelnut Iced Cream* page 338
1 scoop	Vanilla Caramel GNC PM Protein

	Usable Carbs	Fiber	Fat	Protein
Totals for the day (in grams)	18	20	131	192

Simple Menu Planning, Higher Calorie

Day 7

Breakfast

2 pancakes	*Ultralow-Carb Pancakes* page 242
2 cup	Carb Countdown 2% Milk

Snack

2	Hard boiled eggs
1 serving	*Fruity Cottage Cheese* page 270

Lunch

5 wraps	*Spicy Asian Chicken Wraps* page 310
1 serving	*Fat Irish Coffee* page 342

Snack

3 oz	Beef Salami
1 oz	Jarlsberg Cheese

Dinner

2 servings	*Meatloaf* page 288

	Usable Carbs	Fiber	Fat	Protein
Totals for the day (in grams)	15	20	135	194

Simple Menu Planning, Higher Calorie

Day 8

Breakfast

1	*Pepper Cheddar Omelette* page 244
1 scoop	Nectar Fuzzy Navel Protein

Snack

2 wraps	*Spicy Asian Chicken Wraps* page 310
1 serving	Pecans
1 serving	Fat Irish Coffee

Lunch

2 servings	*Meatloaf* page 288
20 nuts	Almonds (about 1/4 of a cup)

Snack

1	Chicken Breast
1 bottle	Carb Countdown Fruit Smoothie

Dinner

1	*Mini-Alfredo Pepperoni & Basil Pizza* page 290
1 scoop	Nectar Roadside Lemonade

Bedtime

1 serving	*Hazelnut Iced Cream* page 338
1 scoop	Vanilla Caramel GNC PM Protein

	Usable Carbs	Fiber	Fat	Protein
Totals for the day (in grams)	13	23	129	203

187

Simple Menu Planning, Higher Calorie

Day 9

Breakfast

6 oz	Ham Steak
1 serving	*Fat Irish Coffee* page 342

Snack

1 link	Chef Bruce Aidells Pesto Sausage
	Mustard for dipping

Lunch

1 serving	*Salmon Teryaki Shaker* page 300
12 nuts	Macadamia

Snack

1 oz	Pepper Jack Cheese
1 bottle	Snapple Diet Iced Tea
1 serving	Colon Cleanse Psyllium Fiber

Dinner

4 servings	*Dijon Chicken Spinach Salad* page 258

Bedtime

1 serving	*Hazelnut Iced Cream* page 338
1 scoop	Vanilla Caramel GNC PM Protein

	Usable Carbs	Fiber	Fat	Protein
Totals for the day (in grams)	5	17	126	192

Simple Menu Planning, Higher Calorie

Day 10

Breakfast

2	*Western Breakfast Wrap* page 250

Lunch

6 slices	Oscar Mayer Ready Serve Bacon
1 scoop	Nectar Fuzzy Navel Protein

It's
Carb Nite!

Gourmet Menu Plans, Lower Calorie

- Require longer preparation
- Greater variety
- More sweets
- Appropriate for 150 lb and below individuals

Items in *italics* can be found in the Recipes section.

Gourmet Menu Planning, Lower Calorie

Day 1

Breakfast

1 serving	*Golden Scrambled Eggs* page 238
2 cookies	*Hazelnut Cookies* page 336
½ scoop	Vanilla Caramel GNC PM Protein

Lunch

5 wraps	*Spicy Asian Chicken Wraps* page 310
1 cup	Coffee + 1 tbsp whipping cream
1 serving	Benefiber

Dinner

2 servings	*Meatloaf* page 288
1 bottle	Carb Countdown Fruit Smoothie
1 serving	Colon Cleanse Psyllium Fiber

	Usable Carbs	Fiber	Fat	Protein
Totals for the day (in grams)	14	15	101	150

Gourmet Menu Planning, Lower Calorie

Day 2

Breakfast

2 pancakes	*Utlra-low Carb Pancakes* page 242
2 slices	Bacon
1 cup	Carb Countdown Chocolate Milk

Lunch

2 servings	*Salmon Cakes* page 298
1 serving	*Lime Dill Sauce* page 318
1 can	Hansen's Diet Soda

Dinner

1 serving	*Salmon Teryaki Shaker* page 300
1 serving	*Pureed Spinach-Turnip Soup* page 256
1 cup	Herbal Tea

	Usable Carbs	Fiber	Fat	Protein
Totals for the day (in grams)	12	13	103	148

Gourmet Menu Planning, Lower Calorie

Day 3

Breakfast

2 serving	*Bacon & Egg Muffin* page 234
1 scone	*Almond Scones* page 232
1 cup	Carb Countdown Skim milk

Lunch

2 servings	*Meatloaf* page 288
2 servings	*Turnip Mashed Potatoes* page 312
1 bottle	Snapple Diet Iced Tea

Dinner

1 serving	*Fish Sticks* page 286
1 scoop	Nectar
1 serving	Colon Cleanse Psyllium Fiber

	Usable Carbs	Fiber	Fat	Protein
Totals for the day (in grams)	18	15	104	153

Gourmet Menu Planning, Lower Calorie

Day 4

Breakfast

2 cakes	*Ricotta Hotcakes* page 246
1 cups	Strawberries, halved
1 cups	Carb Countdown Skim Milk

Lunch

2 servings	*Fish Sticks* page 286
2 servings	*Tartar Sauce* page 322
1 serving	Benefiber

Dinner

1 serving	*Ham Quiche* page 240
1 scoop	GNC PM Protein

	Usable Carbs	Fiber	Fat	Protein
Totals for the day (In grams)	17	10	100	140

Gourmet Menu Planning, Lower Calorie

Day 5

Breakfast

1 serving	*Ham Quiche* page 240
1 scoop	Pure WPI Vanilla Protein Powder
1 cup	Carb Countdown Skim Milk
1 serving	Colon Cleanse Psyllium Fiber

Lunch

1 serving	*Monte Cris-Lo* page 292
1 serving	Benefiber

Dinner

2 servings	*Salmon Cakes* page 298
1 scoop	Nectar

Bedtime

1 serving	*Hazelnut Iced Cream* page 338

	Usable Carbs	Fiber	Fat	Protein
Totals for the day (in grams)	8	9	104	152

Gourmet Menu Planning, Lower Calorie

Day 6

Breakfast

1 serving	*Goat Cheese & Spinach Omelette* page 236
1 scone	*Almond Scones* page 232
1 scoop	WPI Vanilla

Lunch

5 oz	Wild Alaskan Salmon
1 serving	*Creamy Cheese Gelato with Pecans* page 334
1 serving	Benefiber

Dinner

1 serving	*Shellfish & Spinach Bacon Salad* page 260
1 serving	*Pureed Spinach-Turnip Soup* page 256

	Usable Carbs	Fiber	Fat	Protein
Totals for the day (in grams)	18	13	99	142

Gourmet Menu Planning, Lower Calorie

Day 7

Breakfast

2 servings	*Western Breakfast Wraps*	page 250
1 cup	coffee	

Lunch

1 serving	*Mustard fennel Crusted Chicken*	page 296
1 serving	*Dijon Chicken Spinach Salad*	page 258

Dinner

1 serving	*Vegetable Quiche*	page 248
1	Skinless, boneless chicken breast	
1 scoop	Nectar	

Bedtime

1 scoop	GNC PM Protein

	Usable Carbs	Fiber	Fat	Protein
Totals for the day (in grams)	12	22	99	143

Gourmet Menu Planning, Lower Calorie

Day 8

Breakfast

1 serving	*Pepper Cheddar Omelette* page 244
1 serving	Benefiber

Lunch

2 servings	*Deviled Eggs* page 266
2 servings	*Shellfish & Spinach Bacon Salad* page 260

Dinner

4 oz	Turkey breast
1½ serving	*Coconut Cream Pie* page 332

	Usable Carbs	Fiber	Fat	Protein
Totals for the day (in grams)	20	14	100	147

Gourmet Menu Planning, Lower Calorie

Day 9

Breakfast

1 serving	*Vegetable Quiche* page 248
1 scoop	WPI Vanilla
1 cup	Carb Countdown Skim Milk

Lunch

4 oz	Broiled Swordfish
2 cookies	*Hazelnut Cookies* page 336
1 bottle	Snapple Diet Iced Tea
1 serving	Benefiber

Dinner

6 oz	Tri-tip steak
1 serving	*Iced Mocha Latte* page 346

Bedtime

1 scoop	GNC PM Protein

	Usable Carbs	Fiber	Fat	Protein
Totals for the day (in grams)	13	12	96	144

Gourmet Menu Planning, Lower Calorie

Day 10

Breakfast

2 cakes	*Ricotta Hotcakes* page 246
1 cups	Strawberries, halved
1 cups	Carb Countdown Skim Milk

Lunch

3 servings	*Spicy Asian Lettuce Wraps* page 310
1 can	Hansen's Diet Soda

It's

Carb Nite!

Gourmet Menu Plans, Higher Calorie

- Require longer preparation
- Greater variety
- More sweets
- Excellent hunger control
- Appropriate for 150+ lb individuals

Items in *italics* can be found in the Recipes section.

Gourmet Menu Planning, Higher Calorie

Day 1

Breakfast

2 servings	*Bacon & Egg Muffin*	page 234
1 scone	*Almond Scones*	page 232
1 cup	Carb Countdown Skim Milk	
1 scoop	WPI Vanilla	

Snack

3 oz	Smoked Salmon	
1 serving	*Fat Irish Coffee*	page 342

Lunch

2 servings	*Salmon Cakes*	page 298
1 serving	*Lime Dill Sauce*	page 318
1 bottle	Snapple Diet Iced Tea	

Snack

3 oz	Turkey, white meat	
1 bottle	Carb Countdow Fruit Smoothie	

Dinner

6 oz	Tri-tip steak	
1 serving	*Iced Mocha Latte*	page 346

	Usable Carbs	Fiber	Fat	Protein
Totals for the day (in grams)	14	12	136	201

Gourmet Menu Planning, Higher Calorie

Day 2

Breakfast

3 cakes	*Ricotta Hotcakes*	page 246
1 cups	Carb Countdown Skim Milk	

Snack

2 servings	*Bacon & Egg Muffin*	page 234

Lunch

1 serving	*Salmon Teryaki Shaker*	page 300
1 serving	*Simple Spinach Salad*	page 262
1 can	Hansen's Diet Soda	

Snack

2 oz	Cheese stick	
14 slices	*Pepperoni Chips*	page 272

Dinner

1	*Crustless Pizza*	page 284
1 cookie	*Hazelnut Cookies*	page 336
1 bottle	Snapple Diet Iced Tea	
1 serving	Benefiber	

Bedtime

1 scoop	WPI unflavored Protein	
1 cup	Carb Countdown Chocolate Milk	

	Usable Carbs	Fiber	Fat	Protein
Totals for the day (in grams)	17	14	132	198

205

Gourmet Menu Planning, Higher Calorie

Day 3

Breakfast

1 serving	*Golden Scrambled Eggs* page 238	
1 brownie	*Brownies* page 330	
1 cup	Carb Countdown Skim Milk	

Snack

1 scone	*Almond Scones* page 232	
1 cup	Carb Countdown Skim Milk	

Lunch

4 servings	*Dijon Chicken Spinach Salad* page 258	
	Herbal Tea	

Snack

1 serving	*Fruity Cottage Cheese* page 270	

Dinner

1	Chicken Breast	
1 serving	*Roasted Peppers with Garlic & Basil* page 308	

Bedtime

2 servings	*Bacon & Egg Muffin* page 234	
1 scoop	Nectar	

	Usable Carbs	Fiber	Fat	Protein
Totals for the day (in grams)	20	17	131	193

Gourmet Menu Planning, Higher Calorie

Day 4

Breakfast

2 servings	*Western Breakfast Wraps* page 250

Snack

1 serving	*Salmon Cakes* page 298
1 bottle	Snapple Diet Iced Tea

Lunch

1 serving	*Ceasar Tuna Pouch Shaker* page 302
1 scoop	Nectar

Dinner

1 serving	*Vegetable Quiche* page 248
1	Skinless, boneless chicken breast
1 scoop	Nectar

Bedtime

1 serving	*Hazelnut Iced Cream* page 338
1 scoop	Vanilla Caramel GNC PM Protein

	Usable Carbs	Fiber	Fat	Protein
Totals for the day (in grams)	13	21	128	195

Gourmet Menu Planning, Higher Calorie

Day 5

Breakfast

1 serving	*Pepper Cheddar Omelette* page 244
1 cookie	*Almond Butter Cookies* page 328
2 cups	Carb Countdown Skim Milk

Lunch

2 servings	*Fish Sticks* page 286
1 scone	*Almond Scones* page 232
1 serving	*Fat Irish Coffee* page 342

Dinner

2 servings	*Meatloaf* page 288
1 serving	*Turnip Mashed Potatoes* page 312
1 scoop	Nectar Protein Powder

	Usable Carbs	Fiber	Fat	Protein
Totals for the day (in grams)	17	15	137	207

Gourmet Menu Planning, Higher Calorie

Day 6

Breakfast

1 serving	*Ham Quiche* page 240
1 scoop	Pure WPI Vanilla Protein Powder
1 cup	Carb Countdown Skim Milk
¼ cup	Halved Strawberries

Snack

2 wraps	*Spicy Asian Chicken Wraps* page 310
1 bottle	Snapple Diet Iced Tea

Lunch

2 servings	*Meatloaf* page 288
1 serving	*Green Olive Tapénade* page 316
½ serving	*Fat Irish Coffee* page 342

Snack

1 serving	*Shellfish & Spinach Bacon Salad* page 260

Dinner

2 wraps	*Spicy Asian Chicken Wraps* page 310
1 serving	Sugar Free Jello

Bedtime

1 serving	*Hazelnut Iced Cream* page 338
1 scoop	Vanilla Caramel GNC PM Protein

	Usable Carbs	Fiber	Fat	Protein
Totals for the day (in grams)	19	12	126	200

209

Gourmet Menu Planning, Higher Calorie

Day 7

Breakfast

6 oz	Ham Steak
1 serving	*Fat Irish Coffee* page 342

Snack

1 link	Chef Bruce Aidells Artichoke & Garlic Sausage
20 nuts	Pecans
1 scoop	Nectar Protein

Lunch

2 servings	*Mozzarella & Prosciutto Sandwich* page 294
1 scoop	Nectar

Dinner

1	*Mini-Alfredo Pepperoni & Basil Pizza* page 290
3 oz	topped with Chicken
1 can	Hansen's Diet Soda

Bedtime

1 scoop	GNC PM Protein

	Usable Carbs	Fiber	Fat	Protein
Totals for the day (in grams)	15	21	131	194

Gourmet Menu Planning, Higher Calorie

Day 8

Breakfast

1 serving	*Goat Cheese & Spinach Omelette* page 236
3 oz	Ham Steak
1 serving	*Fat Irish Coffee* page 342

Lunch

4 servings	*Dijon Chicken Spinach Salad* page 258
1 serving	Sugar-Free Jello

Dinner

2	*Chicken Fajitas* page 282
1 bottle	Snapple Diet Iced Tea

Bedtime

1 serving	*Coconut Cream Pie* page 332
1 cup	Carb Countdown Skim Milk
1 scoop	WPI Vanilla Protein

	Usable Carbs	Fiber	Fat	Protein
Totals for the day (in grams)	19	26	133	196

Gourmet Menu Planning, Higher Calorie

Day 9

Breakfast

4	Fried Eggs
3 oz	Canadian Bacon
1 serving	*Fat Irish Coffee* page 342

Snack

1 serving	*Mozzarella & Prosciutto Sandwich* page 294

Lunch

1 serving	*Monte Cris-Lo* page 292
1 can	Hansen's Diet Soda

Snack

1 serving	*Shellfish & Spinach Bacon Salad* page 260

Dinner

1 serving	*Bell Pepper Tacos* page 278
1 serving	Sugar Free Jello

	Usable Carbs	Fiber	Fat	Protein
Totals for the day (in grams)	15	12	136	195

Gourmet Menu Planning, Higher Calorie

Day 10

Breakfast

6 oz	Ham Steak
1 oz	Colby Cheese

Snack

1 serving	*Fruity Cottage Cheese* page 270
35 nuts	Almonds (about 1/3 of a cup)

Lunch

1 serving	*Ham Quiche* page 240

It's
Carb Nite!

Example Carb Nites

Sample Carb Nites

Example 1

4:00 PM

All natural granola

Yogurt

6:00 PM

Homemade biscuits with jelly

Grilled catfish

Mashed potatoes

Peas

Peach cobbler with vanilla ice cream

9:00 PM

Cookies

Warm glass of milk

Sample Carb Nites

Example 2

6:00 PM

Breadsticks

Pizza

Maybe a few spicy buffalo wings

Blueberry pie ala mode

9:00 PM

Chocolate covered pretzels

Rice pudding

Sample Carb Nites

Example 3

5:00 PM

    Hamburger with fries

    Oreo® Milkshake

    Key lime pie

8:30 PM

    Peanut butter and jelly sandwich

    Milk

Midnight

    Dark chocolate covered almonds

Sample Carb Nites

Example 4

4:30 PM

Decaffe Latte with whipped cream

Lemon poppyseed poundcake

7:00 PM

Faccocia bread with olive oil

Lasagna

Meatballs

New York style cheesecake

9:30 PM

Donuts

Transition Menu Plan

- Use when ending The Carb Nite Solution
- Reduces carb-rebound effect
- Preserves fat accelerated fat burning
- Appropriate for all users

Items in *italics* can be found in the Recipes section.

Four Day Transition Plan for Ending The Solution

Day 1

Breakfast

4	Fried Eggs
2 oz	Canadian Bacon

Lunch

5 servings	*Spicy Asian Lettuce Wraps* page 310

Mini-Carb Nite

Dinner

¾ cup	Tortellini Pasta with Marinara sauce

Bedtime

1 cup	French Vanilla Ice Cream

Four Day Transition Plan for Ending The Solution

Day 2

Breakfast

6 oz	Ham Steak
1 oz	Colby Cheese
2	Hard-boiled eggs

Lunch

2 links	Chef Bruce Aidells Habanero & Green Chili Sausage
1 oz	Cheddar Cheese
	Mustard to taste

Mini-Carb Nite

Dinner

1	Chicken breast
1 cup	Long grain wild rice
1 cup	Mixed vegetables

Bedtime

1 serving	Peach cobbler

Four Day Transition Plan for Ending The Solution

Day 3

Breakfast

2 pancakes	*Ultralow-Carb Pancakes* page 242
1 cup	Carb Countdown 2% Milk
3 slices	Oscar Mayer Ready Serve Bacon

Lunch

1 serving	*Ranch Tuna Pouch Shaker* page 302
1 tbsp	Real Bacon Bits

Mini-Carb Nite

Dinner

3 oz	Turkey
1 cup	Mashed Potatoes
1 cup	Mixed Vegetables

Bedtime

1 piece	Chocolate Cake

Four Day Transition Plan for Ending The Solution

Day 4

Breakfast

1	*Goat Cheese & Spinach Omelette* page 236
1 cup	Carb Countdown Skim Milk

Lunch

1 serving	*Ceasar Tuna Pouch Shaker* page 302
2 oz	Jarlsberg Cheese

Mini-Carb Nite

Dinner

1	Ham Sandwich
1 cup	Potato Salad

Bedtime

3	Cookies

Recipes

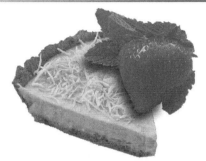

Ultralow-Carb Coconut Cream Pie
with toasted coconut
and strawberry

Breakfast

Savory Crust

What to gather

1 ½ cups	Hazelnut meal
2 tbsp	Butter, chilled
2 tbsp	Heavy whipping cream
	Salt
	Black pepper

prep: basic

How to prepare

In a food processor, blend all ingredients until dough is combined and clumps together. Chill for 15 minutes.

Press dough into an 8" nonstick pie pan and bake at 325° for 10 minutes.

Almond Scones

What to gather

1	Egg
1	Egg white
⅓ cup	Almond oil
⅓ cup	Splenda for baking
⅓ cup	Heavy whipping cream
⅓ cup	Philadelphia whipped cream cheese
1 tsp	Vanilla extract
1 cup	GNC PM Protein, vanilla caramel flavor
1 cup	Almond meal
1 tsp	Baking powder
½ tsp	Baking soda
½ cup	Toasted almond slices

Almond Scones

How to prepare

Preheat oven to 325°F.

Spray cookie sheet with nonstick cooking spray.

In large mixing bowl, blend egg and egg white. Add almond oil, Splenda, whipping cream, cream cheese and vanilla until cream cheese breaks down.

In a separate bowl, mix protein powder, almond meal, baking powder, baking soda and almonds. Blend dry ingredients into wet ingredients until combined.

Mound 12 spoonfuls of batter on prepared baking sheet.

Bake 10 to 15 minutes or until lightly golden brown.

Nutrition Facts per Serving

Usable Carbs	Fiber	Fat	Protein	Score
2	2	19	9	F

Bacon & Egg Muffins

What to gather

2 tsp	Olive oil
5 oz	Morel mushrooms, chopped
6 slices	Bacon
4	Eggs
½ cup	Carb Countdown 2% Milk
1 tbsp	Grain mustard
1 tbsp	Flat-leaf parsley, roughly chopped
½ tsp	Sea salt
¼ cup	Cheddar cheese, grated

How to prepare

Preheat oven to 300°F.

Heat frying pan over medium-high heat. Add oil and mushrooms and cook for 5 minutes or until mushrooms are soft and golden. Remove mixture from pan and set aside.

Add the bacon to pan and cook for 5 minutes or until golden.

Grease six 4 oz capacity muffin tins with oil. Cut bacon to fit the inside of each muffin hole (using the wider end around the side and the tail of the bacon to line the bottom).

Whisk together the eggs, milk, grain mustard, parsley and salt. Divide the mushrooms and cheese between muffin tins and top with the egg mixture.

Bake for 25 minutes or until golden. Serve warm or cold.

Nutrition Facts per Serving

Usable Carbs	Fiber	Fat	Protein	Score
0	1	7	7	N

Goat Cheese & Spinach Omelette

What to gather

3	Eggs
2 oz	Chevre cheese
1 cup	Baby spinach, fresh
¼	Bell pepper
1 tsp	Butter

Goat Cheese & Spinach Omelette

prep: basic

How to prepare

In a small non-stick skillet over medium heat, melt butter.

In a small bowl, scramble eggs and pour into skillet. Without stirring, let eggs firm up around the edges and flip eggs over. Immediately place cheese, spinach and peppers on eggs and fold omelette in half.

Remove from heat and transfer omelette to serving plate. Serve immediately.

Nutrition Facts per Serving

Usable Carbs	Fiber	Fat	Protein	Score
3	1	29	28	N

Golden Scrambled Eggs

What to gather

2	Whole eggs
2	Egg whites
1 tsp	Butter

prep: basic

How to prepare

In a small non-stick skillet over medium heat, melt butter.

In a small mixing bowl, whisk egg whites and whole eggs until combined. Pour eggs into skillet.

Using a heat resistant spatula continually scrape the bottom of the pan to scramble eggs until light and fluffy, approximately 4-5 minutes. Serve warm.

Nutrition Facts per Serving

Usable Carbs	Fiber	Fat	Protein	Score
1	0	14	20	N

Ham Quiche

What to gather

1	Savory Crust, prepared page 230
2 tbsp	Olive oil
1 cup	Smoked ham, diced
½ small	Red bell pepper
6 large	Eggs
½ cup	Heavy whipping cream
	Salt
	Black pepper

How to prepare

Preheat oven to 350°.

Prepare piecrust in an 8″ pie pan.

In a frying pan, sauté ham and bell pepper in olive oil until bell pepper has wilted. Remove from heat.

In a medium sized mixing bowl, beat eggs until frothy and then mix in cream. Season egg mixture with salt and pepper.

Arrange ham and bell peppers over the bottom of prepared pie crust and carefully pour in egg mixture: the filling should be about one inch from the top of the pie pan.

Bake for 30–35 minutes or until quiche is golden brown and puffy. Cool for 20 minutes before serving.

Nutrition Facts per Serving

Usable Carbs	Fiber	Fat	Protein	Score
3	2	32	11	F+

Pancakes

What to gather

1 scoop	GNC PM Protein, vanilla caramel flavor
½ tsp	Vanilla extract
½ tsp	Almond extract
2 scoop	Whole eggs
1 tbsp	Canola oil
1 tbsp	Pure psyllium fiber
2 tbsp	Water
½ tbsp	Butter
1 tbsp	Water

prep: basic

How to prepare

In a small mixing bowl, whisk all ingredients except for butter until smooth.

In a small skillet over medium-high heat, melt half of butter while swirling around the pan to coat bottom.

Pour half of batter into skillet and cook for 2-3 minutes or until edges of pancake begin to brown. Flip pancake and cook for one more minute. Transfer pancake to a plate.

Repeat for remaining batter.

Nutrition Facts per Serving

Usable Carbs	Fiber	Fat	Protein	Score
1	3	14	16	N

Pepper Cheddar Omelette

What to gather

2	Eggs
2 oz	Cheddar cheese, shredded
1 medium	Banana pepper, sliced
½ tsp	Butter

Pepper Cheddar Omelette

prep: basic

How to prepare

In a small non-stick skillet over medium heat, melt butter.

In a small bowl, scramble eggs and pour into skillet. Without stirring, let eggs firm up around the edges and flip eggs over. Immediately place cheese and peppers on eggs and fold omelette in half.

Remove from heat and transfer omelette to a plate. Serve immediately.

Nutrition Facts per Serving

Usable Carbs	Fiber	Fat	Protein	Score
2	2	32	27	F

Ricotta Hotcakes

What to gather

4 oz	Ricotta cheese
2 tbsp	Heavy whipping cream
2	Eggs, separated
1 scoop	GNC PM Protein, vanilla caramel flavor
1 tbsp	Pure psyllium fiber
½ tsp	Baking powder
dash	Cinnamon
dash	Salt
1 tbsp	Water
1 tsp	Vanilla extract
1 tbsp	Butter

prep: basic

How to prepare

In a small mixing bowl, whisk ricotta cheese, heavy whipping cream, and egg yolks. Add protein powder, psyllium fiber, baking powder, cinnamon, salt and water until thoroughly combined and smooth. Set aside.

In a small bowl, whisk egg whites until foamy. Fold egg whites and vanilla with a spoon or spatula into batter.

In a large skillet over medium-high heat, melt one third of butter and swirl around to coat the bottom of the pan. Pour one third of batter into skillet and cook for 3-4 minutes or until the edges of the hotcakes begin to brown. Flip hotcake and cook for 2-3 more minutes. Transfer pancake to a plate.

Repeat for remaining batter.

Nutrition Facts per Serving

Usable Carbs	Fiber	Fat	Protein	Score
2	2	17	15	F

Vegetable Quiche

What to gather

1	Savory Crust, prepared page 230
2 tbsp	Olive oil
2 cups	Baby spinach, fresh
3 medium	Banana peppers, seeds removed, diced
1 cup	Chanterelle mushrooms, sliced
½ cup	Feta cheese, crumbled
6 large	Eggs
½ cup	Heavy whipping cream
	Salt
	Pepper

prep: moderate

How to prepare

Preheat oven to 350°F.

In a large frying pan, sauté spinach, peppers and mushrooms in olive oil until mushrooms brown and spinach wilts. Remove from heat and set aside.

In a medium sized mixing bowl, beat eggs until frothy and then mix in cream. Season egg mixture with salt and pepper.

Arrange spinach, peppers and mushrooms over the bottom of prepared piecrust. Scatter goat cheese over vegetables. Carefully pour in egg mixture: the filling should be about one inch from the top of the pie pan.

Bake in oven for 30-35 minutes or until quiche is golden brown and puffy. Cool for 20 minutes before serving.

Nutrition Facts per Serving

Usable Carbs	Fiber	Fat	Protein	Score
3	4	33	10	F+

Western Breakfast Wraps

What to gather

1 tsp	Butter
2 oz	Ham, diced
2 large	Eggs, beaten
1 oz	Cheddar cheese, shredded
2	Low-carb tortilla shells

How to prepare

In a small nonstick skillet over medium-high heat, melt butter. Add ham and cook until ham begins to brown, approximately 3-4 minutes. Reduce heat to medium and add beaten egg. Cook another 2-3 minutes.

Spoon half the egg and ham mixture down the center of a single tortilla shell, top with cheddar cheese, roll up and serve.

Repeat for remaining tortilla shell.

Nutrition Facts per Serving

Usable Carbs	Fiber	Fat	Protein	Score
4	8	17	21	N

Soups & Salads

Creamy Turnip-Cheese Soup

What to gather

2 tbsp	Butter
1 large	Garlic clove, peeled and minced
3 medium	Turnips, peeled and chopped
2 cups	Chicken stock
¼ cup	Cream cheese
1½ cup	Carb Countdown 2% milk
4 oz	Sharp cheddar cheese
	Salt
	Black pepper

prep: moderate

How to prepare

In a medium pot over medium heat, melt butter. Add garlic and cook, stirring often for 5 minutes. Add turnips and cook, stirring often, until turnips are soft, 6-8 minutes. Add stock and simmer for 15 minutes.

In blender, working in batches, puree stock mixture with cream cheese and Carb Countdown until smooth. Return soup to pot, over medium heat.

Whisk in cheddar, stirring until soup is hot and smooth.

Season to taste with salt and pepper and serve.

Nutrition Facts per Serving

Usable Carbs	Fiber	Fat	Protein	Score
3	1	11	7	F

Pureed Spinach-Turnip Soup

What to gather

1 tbsp	Butter
2 medium	Garlic cloves, peeled and minced
½ lb	Turnips, peeled and cubed
2 cups	Chicken stock
1 bunch	Baby spinach, stems removed
	Salt
	Black pepper

How to prepare

In a large saucepan over medium heat, melt butter. Add garlic, and turnips; stir to coat. Cook 2 minutes while continuing to stir. Pour chicken broth and 1/2 cup water into pan; stir to combine. Bring to a boil. Reduce heat to medium-low, cover and simmer until turnips are very tender, about 12 minutes. Stir spinach into pan, and cook until wilted and bright green, about 3 minutes. Remove from heat.

In blender, working in batches, puree soup until smooth.

Season with salt and pepper, and serve.

Nutrition Facts per Serving

Usable Carbs	Fiber	Fat	Protein	Score
6	5	7	6	F

Dijon Chicken Spinach Salad

What to gather

2 handfuls	Baby spinach
6 oz	Diced chicken, white meat
5 tbsp	Red wine vinegar
1 tsp	Dijon mustard
2 tbsp	Olive oil
2 tbsp	Parmesan cheese, grated
1 clove	Garlic, minced
	Salt
	Black pepper

Dijon Chicken Spinach Salad

prep: basic

How to prepare

In a medium bowl, place spinach and chicken; set aside.

In a small bowl, whisk the vinegar and mustard and slowly add the olive oil until emulsified, then add garlic, salt and pepper.

Pour dressing over spinach and mix well with a fork.

Nutrition Facts per Serving

Usable Carbs	Fiber	Fat	Protein	Score
0	1	9	14	N

Shellfish & Spinach Bacon Salad

What to gather

2	slices	Bacon, thick
2	cloves	Garlic, minced
¼	cup	Chicken stock
⅛	tsp	Crushed red pepper
¾	lb	Fresh scallops
12	oz	Baby spinach

How to prepare

In a Dutch oven over medium heat, cook bacon until crisp. Remove bacon, retaining drippings in pan. Crumble bacon and set aside.

Add garlic to drippings in pan; cook over medium heat 1 minute. Add vegetable stock and crushed red pepper. Add scallops to pan; cook 3-4 minutes; turn scallops over and cook another 3-4 minutes. Remove scallops from heat; set aside.

Add spinach to stock mixture in pan; cook 1 minute or until spinach wilts. Divide spinach mixture between 2 medium bowls; sprinkle evenly with bacon. Arrange scallops over the spinach mixture; drizzle evenly with any remaining stock mixture.

Nutrition Facts per Serving

Usable Carbs	Fiber	Fat	Protein	Score
6	2	8	35	P

Simple Spinach Salad

What to gather

1 cup	Baby spinach
½ tbsp	Olive Oil
1½ tbsp	Rice vinegar, unflavored
	Salt
	Black pepper

prep: basic

How to prepare

In a small bowl, drizzle olive oil and vinegar over spinach and toss with a fork.

Season with salt and pepper to taste.

Nutrition Facts per Serving

Usable Carbs	Fiber	Fat	Protein	Score
0	0	7	0	F+

Snacks

Deviled Eggs

What to gather

2	Hardboiled eggs
1 tbsp	Saffola Mayonnaise
1 tsp	Mustard
1 tbsp	Cheddar cheese, grated
	Paprika
	Black pepper

Deviled Eggs

prep: basic

How to prepare

Peel hard-boiled eggs and discard shells. Cut eggs down the center length-wise and remove yolks. In a small bowl, mix egg yolks, mayonnaise, mustard and pepper until smooth and creamy. Mix in cheese. Fill each egg white with one tablespoon of filling and sprinkle with paprika. Serve chilled.

Nutrition Facts per Serving

Usable Carbs	Fiber	Fat	Protein	Score
0	0	6	2	F+

Egg Salad Wrap

What to gather

1	Low-carb tortilla shell
2 tbsp	Celery, chopped
1 tbsp	Saffola Mayonnaise
1 tsp	Chopped dill, fresh
1 tsp	Whole grain mustard
1 tsp	Lime juice
½ tsp	Kosher salt
1 large	Hardboiled egg, chopped
	Black pepper

Egg Salad Wrap

How to prepare

In a medium bowl, mix together celery, mayonnaise, dill, mustard, lime juice and salt. Gently fold in chopped egg. Season to taste with freshly ground black pepper. Spoon egg mixture down the center of tortilla shell; roll up and serve.

Nutrition Facts per Serving

Usable Carbs	Fiber	Fat	Protein	Score
5	8	18	11	F

Fruity Cottage Cheese

What to gather

½ cup	Cottage cheese
1 tbsp	Heavy whipping cream
½ tbsp	Torani sugar-free peach syrup
1 tbsp	Benefiber

Fruity Cottage Cheese

How to prepare

In a small bowl, combine all ingredients with a spoon. Serve chilled. Substitute peach syrup with your favorite sugar-free fruit flavored syrup.

Nutrition Facts per Serving

Usable Carbs	Fiber	Fat	Protein	Score
3	3	11	13	N

Pepperoni Chips

What to gather

14 slices   Hormel pepperoni, sliced

Pepperoni Chips

How to prepare

On microwave safe plate, layer two paper towels on top of each other. Arrange pepperoni slices on paper towels, being careful to avoid any overlap. Cover with two more paper towels. Microwave on high power for 1 to 1½ minutes; rotate plate. Microwave for another 1 to 1½ minutes. Remove plate from microwave and immediately press down firmly and evenly on paper towel layers. Remove top two paper towels and move pepperoni chips to clean dish. Cool at least 1 minute before eating.

Several batches can be made and stored for convenient snacking.

Nutrition Facts per Serving

Usable Carbs	Fiber	Fat	Protein	Score
0	0	1	5	P

Entrees

Breadcrumb Substitute

What to gather

6 oz   Pork rinds

Breadcrumb Substitute

How to prepare

Fill food processor with whole pork rinds. Process until finely ground and fluffy.

Remove pork rind crumbs from processor and place in air-tight storage container.

Repeat for remainder of bag.

Bell Pepper Tacos

servings: 2

What to gather

½ lb	Ground beef, extra lean
2 tbsp	Canola oil
½ package	Taco seasoning, low-carb
1 large	Green bell pepper
½ cup	Cheddar cheese, shredded
2 tbsp	Jalapenos, diced

Bell Pepper Tacos

How to prepare

In a medium non-stick heavy skillet, brown ground beef. Drain extra fat drippings and discard. Return skillet to burner and reduce heat to low. Add oil and taco seasoning until well combined. Remove from heat.

Slice bell pepper lengthwise and discard stems, ribs and seeds. Stuff half of the meat mixture in each side of a bell pepper and top with cheddar cheese and jalapenos. Serve warm.

Nutrition Facts per Serving

Usable Carbs	Fiber	Fat	Protein	Score
3	2	32	47	N

Broiled Salmon with Feta

What to gather

1 tsp	Olive oil
6 oz	Wild Alaskan salmon, fresh
½ tbsp	No carb seafood seasoning blend
¼ cup	Feta cheese, crumbled
½ tsp	Sun dried tomatoes, diced

Broiled Salmon with Feta

How to prepare

Turn oven to Broil.

On broiling pan, place salmon and brush with olive oil. Sprinkle seasoning blend on top of salmon and broil fish for 10-12 minutes. Remove from oven and top with feta cheese and sun dried tomatoes. Serve immediately.

Nutrition Facts per Serving

Usable Carbs	Fiber	Fat	Protein	Score
2	0	33	51	N

Chicken Fajitas

What to gather

3 oz	Chicken breast, precooked
½ small	Green bell pepper
2 oz	Cheddar cheese, shredded
2 tbsp	Sour cream
2 tbsp	Mild hot sauce
1 tbsp	Low-carb tomato and basil pasta sauce
¼ cup	Iceburg lettuce, shredded
2	Low-carb tortillas

prep: basic

How to prepare

On cookie sheet, arrange tortilla shells and warm in 200°F oven, 2-3 minutes or microwave tortillas for 30 seconds on high.

Cut chicken breast into finger-sized strips. In a heavy non-stick skillet over medium-high heat, brown chicken strips until tender; add peppers to skillet and sauté for 30 seconds. Remove chicken and peppers from heat.

Down the center of one tortilla shell stack half of the chicken strips, peppers, cheese, sour cream, hot sauce, pasta sauce and lettuce; roll the edges of the tortilla shell around the filling. Repeat for second tortilla shell.

Nutrition Facts per Serving

Usable Carbs	Fiber	Fat	Protein	Score
4	8	16	26	N

Crustless Pizza

What to gather

34 slices	Hormel turkey pepperoni
¼ cup	Mozzarella cheese, shredded
2 tbsp	Low-carb pasta sauce

Crustless Pizza

How to prepare

On a microwave safe plate, arrange pepperoni slices in circular fashion, starting on the outer rim and moving inward, to form the bottom of pizza. Sprinkle pepperoni layer with tomato sauce. Spread cheese on top. Microwave for 3 to 3½ minutes on medium power. Remove from microwave; let stand 2 minutes before serving.

Nutrition Facts per Serving

Usable Carbs	Fiber	Fat	Protein	Score
2	0	14	25	N

Fish Sticks

What to gather

2 cups	Breadcrumb substitute page 276
½ cup	Parmesan cheese, grated
	Salt
	Black pepper
2	Whole eggs
1 lb	Cod

prep: moderate

How to prepare

Preheat oven to 350°.

In a bowl, mix together breadcrumb substitute, parmesan cheese and pepper. Pour mixture onto a plate.

In a bowl, whisk together eggs.

Cut cod filets into finger-sized strips. Coat strips with egg by dipping into egg wash. Follow by rolling fish stick in breadcrumb and cheese mixture. Place on a greased baking sheet. Repeat with remaining finger-sized strips.

Bake coated fish fingers in oven for 25-30 minutes or until fish is flaky and crust is golden brown.

Enjoy with tartar sauce, page 322.

Nutrition Facts per Serving

Usable Carbs	Fiber	Fat	Protein	Score
1	0	11	33	P

Meatloaf

What to gather

2 lbs	Extra lean ground beef
2	Eggs
¼ cup	Parmesan cheese, grated
1 small	Green bell pepper
⅓ cup	Hazelnut meal
¼ cup	Low-carb ketchup
4 tbsp	Canola oil
1 tbsp	Dijon mustard
1 tbsp	Garlic, minced
½ tsp	Oregano
1 tsp	Salt
1 tsp	Black pepper

prep: basic

How to prepare

Preheat oven to 350°F.

In a large bowl, combine all ingredients and stir until well mixed. Place mixture in an 8" by 4" loaf pan coated with non-stick cooking spray.

Bake meat loaf for 40-45 minutes. Let stand for 10 minutes and serve.

Nutrition Facts per Serving

Usable Carbs	Fiber	Fat	Protein	Score
0	0	16	29	N

Mini Alfredo, Pepperoni & Basil Pizza

What to gather

4 leaves	Fresh basil
2 tbsp	Low-carb puttanesca pasta sauce
2 tbsp	Low-carb Alfredo sauce
1 oz	Pepperoni, sliced (about 12-14 slices)
½ cup	Mozzarella cheese, shredded
1	Low-carb tortilla shell

Mini Alfredo, Pepperoni & Basil Pizza

prep: basic

How to prepare

Conventional oven (for crispy crust):

Preheat oven to 325°F.

On a nonstick baking sheet, lie tortilla shell flat and top with marinara and Alfredo sauces, spreading evenly. Follow with pepperoni and basil leaves. Top with mozzarella cheese.

Bake for 10-12 minutes or until cheese is bubbly. Serve warm.

Microwave oven:

On microwave-safe plate, prepare pizza in same manner as above. Microwave on med-high power for 3 minutes. Let stand 2 minutes before serving.

Nutrition Facts per Serving

Usable Carbs	Fiber	Fat	Protein	Score
6	8	25	14	F

Monte Cris-Lo

What to gather

6 oz   Pastrami

2 oz   Jarlsberg or Swiss cheese

¼ cup Sauerkraut

1 tbsp Stone-ground mustard

prep: basic

How to prepare

Turn oven to broil and raise the top rack to highest level.

In a shallow baking dish, broil pastrami until the edges start to brown or about 5 minutes. You may also use a toaster oven set to broil. Remove pastrami from oven, top with Jarlsberg or Swiss cheese and broil for one minute more.

Remove from oven and top with sourkraut and mustard. Serve immediately.

Nutrition Facts per Serving

Usable Carbs	Fiber	Fat	Protein	Score
1	1	24	50	N

Mozzarella & Prosciutto Sandwich

What to gather

6 oz	Mozzarella ball
6 oz	Prosciutto ham
6 leaves	Basil, fresh
¾ cup	Hazelnut meal
1	Egg
1 tbsp	Butter
1 tsp	Olive oil
	Salt
	Black pepper

Mozzarella & Prosciutto Sandwich

How to prepare

In a small bowl, beat egg; set aside.

On plate, poor hazelnut meal and add salt and pepper. Spread evenly.

In a large skillet over medium heat, warm butter and olive oil.

Cut mozzarella ball into 12 thin slices. Dip one side of the mozzarella slice into egg wash and then into hazelnut meal and place battered side down on hot skillet. Stack one large slice of prosciutto and 2 fresh basil leaves on top of the mozzarella. Dip another slice of mozzarella in egg wash and hazelnut meal and place battered side up on top of basil. Cook for 1 – 2 minutes. Flip sandwich and cook for one more minute or until golden brown. Place on plate and serve immediately.

Nutrition Facts per Serving

Usable Carbs	Fiber	Fat	Protein	Score
3	2	25	17	F

Mustard-Fennel Crusted Chicken

What to gather

8	Chicken thighs, bone-in with skin
3 tbsp	Extra virgin olive oil
1 tbsp	Fennel seeds
1 cup	Breadcrumb substitute page 276
2 tbsp	Dijon mustard
2 tbsp	Parsley, chopped
	Salt
	Black pepper

Mustard-Fennel Crusted Chicken

prep: place 911 on speed-dial

How to prepare

Set a rack in the center of the oven and heat the oven to 400°F.

Rinse the chicken parts and pat them dry; season generously with salt and pepper. Heat 1 tbsp of oil in a 10-inch sauté pan over medium-high heat until hot. Brown the chicken well on both sides, 3-4 minutes per side. Transfer the chicken, skin side up, to a 1″ by 14″ or similar roasting pan and bake until cooked through, about 15 minutes.

Meanwhile, in a small dry skillet over medium heat, toast the fennel seeds, stirring frequently, until golden and fragrant, about 2-3 minutes. Transfer to a small bowl and add remaining olive oil, breadcrumb substitute, salt and pepper.

Remove the chicken from the oven and raise oven temperature to 500°F. Turn the chicken pieces over and lightly dab with mustard using pastry brush. Press seasoned pork rind mixture on top of the mustard. Bake until the crust turns golden brown, about another 10 minutes. Transfer the chicken to a serving platter, sprinkle with parsley and serve.

Nutrition Facts per Serving

Usable Carbs	Fiber	Fat	Protein	Score
0	0	17	19	N

Salmon Cakes

What to gather

3 tbsp	Butter
1	Green onion, finely chopped
⅛ cup	Red bell pepper, finely chopped
2 cloves	Garlic, minced
3 tbsp	Heavy whipping cream
1 tbsp	Dijon mustard
1	Egg
½ tsp	Parsley, minced
	Cayenne pepper
1 cup	Breadcrumb substitute page 276
¼ cup	Parmesan cheese, grated
1 lb	Wild Alaskan salmon, chopped
2 tbsp	Olive oil

Salmon Cakes

How to prepare

In a large skillet over medium heat, melt 1 tbsp butter. Sauté onion, bell pepper and garlic until the pepper is limp, about 3 minutes. Add the cream, mustard, egg, parsley, cayenne pepper and ½ cup breadcrumb substitute. Remove from heat. Gently fold in salmon.

Form the mixture into 8 patties, about ½ an inch thick. In a mixing bowl, combine the remaining ½ cup of breadcrumb substitute with parmesan cheese. Pat this topping onto both sides of the patties. Refrigerate for 2 hours.

In a large skillet over medium-high heat combine the oil and remaining 2 tablespoons of butter. Sauté the crab cakes in the hot oil-butter mixture for about 3 minutes on each side or until golden brown.

Enjoy with lime-dill sauce, page 318.

Nutrition Facts per Serving

Usable Carbs	Fiber	Fat	Protein	Score
0	0	20	22	N

Salmon Teriyaki Shaker

What to gather

7 oz   Chicken of the Sea pink salmon pouch

2 tbsp Carb Option Asian Teriyaki Sauce

prep: basic

How to prepare

In a quart-sized container (such as a quart sized Ziploc® bag), combine all ingredients and seal container. Shake until well combined.

Nutrition Facts per Serving

Usable Carbs	Fiber	Fat	Protein	Score
0	0	9	49	P

Tuna Pouch Shakers

What to gather

3 oz   Tuna pouch

2 tbsp Low-carb Ranch or Ceasar dressing

1 oz   Parmesan cheese, grated (about ¼ cup)

¼ tbsp Canola oil

prep: basic

How to prepare

In a quart-sized container (such as a quart sized Ziploc bag), combine all ingredients and seal container. Shake until well combined.

Nutrition Facts per Serving

Usable Carbs	Fiber	Fat	Protein	Score
1	0	26	33	N

Side Dishes

Classic Turnip Salad

What to gather

1½ lbs	Turnips
¼ cup	Celery, finely chopped
3 spears	Kosher dill pickles
2 large	Hardboiled eggs, chopped
⅓ cup	Saffola Mayonnaise
2 tbsp	Rice vinegar, unflavored
1 tbsp	Dijon Mustard
¼ tsp	Sea salt
¼ tsp	Black pepper, freshly ground

Classic Turnip Salad

How to prepare

Preheat oven to 400°F.

Pierce turnips with a fork and wrap each turnip separately in tin foil. Bake turnips for 25 minutes or until tender when pierced with a fork. Remove from oven and let stand until completely cooled.

Using a clean, dry paper towel, rub turnips to remove skins. Cut turnips in ½-inch cubes. Combine turnips, celery, pickles and eggs in a large bowl.

In a small bowl, whisk mayonnaise and remaining ingredients until combined. Pour over turnip mixture, tossing gently to coat. Cover and refrigerate for at least 4 hours.

Nutrition Facts per Serving

Usable Carbs	Fiber	Fat	Protein	Score
5	2	17	4	F+

Roasted Bell Peppers

What to gather

4 medium	Green bell peppers
¼ cup	Olive oil
1 tbsp	White wine vinegar
2 cloves	Garlic, halved
4 leaves	Basil, de-stemmed
	Salt
	Black pepper

Roasted Bell Peppers

How to prepare

Heat broiler, with rack 6 inches from top heat.

Cut peppers in half through the stem; discard stems, ribs, and seeds. On a rimmed baking sheet, place peppers cut side down.

Roast peppers under the broiler until skins are charred, rotating baking sheet occasionally to cook evenly, about 10 minutes. Transfer peppers to bowl, and cover with plastic wrap. Let steam until cool enough to handle, about 10 minutes.

Using a clean, dry paper towel, rub peppers to remove blackened skin. Cut peppers into strips, and return to bowl. Add oil, vinegar, garlic, and basil; season with salt and pepper. Toss to combine. Serve warm or at room temperature.

Nutrition Facts per Serving

Usable Carbs	Fiber	Fat	Protein	Score
4	2	14	0	F+

Spicy Asian Lettuce Wraps

What to gather

¼ cup	Cilantro, fresh
¼ cup	Soy sauce
1 tbsp	Chili paste with garlic
2 tbsp	Sesame oil, dark
2 cups	Boneless, skinless chicken breast, diced
10 leaves	Romaine lettuce, outermost leaves

How to prepare

In a large bowl, whisk cilantro, soy sauce, chili paste and oil. Add chicken to soy mixture; toss well to coat.

Spoon about ⅓ cup chicken mixture down center of each lettuce leaf; roll up and serve.

Nutrition Facts per Serving

Usable Carbs	Fiber	Fat	Protein	Score
1	1	4	9	P

Turnip Mashed Potatoes

What to gather

2 medium Turnips

⅓ cup   Whipped cream cheese

1½ tbsp   Butter

1 tsp   Garlic powder

½ tsp   Onion salt

½ tsp   Cream of tartar

         Salt

         Black pepper

Turnip Mashed Potatoes

prep: moderate

How to prepare

Preheat oven to 350°F.

Wrap each turnip in tin foil and bake for 30 minutes or until a fork inserts easily into turnip. Using a fork, carefully remove skins from hot turnips; discard skins.

In a food processor, mix turnips, cream cheese, butter and seasonings until thick and smooth. Pour into glass serving bowl and serve immediately.

Nutrition Facts per Serving

Usable Carbs	Fiber	Fat	Protein	Score
5	3	11	2	F+

Sauces, Spreads & Dips

Green Olive Tapénade

What to gather

2 cups	Green olives with pimientos
2 tbsp	Capers
7	Anchovy fillets, marinated
1 tsp	Lemon zest
1 tsp	Parsley, finely chopped
½ cup	Olive oil

prep: basic

How to prepare

In food processor, puree all ingredients except olive oil. Add olive oil and pulse until incorporated.

Nutrition Facts per Serving (approx ⅓ cup)

Usable Carbs	Fiber	Fat	Protein	Score
0	0	17	1	F+

Lime Dill Sauce

What to gather

1 cup	Saffola Mayonnaise
2 tbsp	Dill leaves, finely chopped
1 tbsp	Parsley leaves, finely chopped
1 tbsp	Lime zest, grated
2 tbsp	Lime juice
1 clove	Garlic, minced

Lime Dill Sauce

prep: basic

How to prepare

In a small bowl, combine all ingredients together until well blended. Chill at least 2 hours before serving.

Nutrition Facts per Serving (approx 1 tbsp)

Usable Carbs	Fiber	Fat	Protein	Score
0	0	9	0	F+

Lime Caper Mayonnaise

What to gather

2	Egg yolks
1¼ cups	Canola oil
1 tsp	Lime juice
1 tbsp	Capers
pinch	Sea salt

Lime Caper Mayonnaise

How to prepare

In a small bowl, whisk egg yolks and slowly add the olive oil until emulsified. Add lime juice. As mixture thickens, add capers and salt. Leave in serving bowl for dipping.

Nutrition Facts per Serving (approx 1 tbsp)

Usable Carbs	Fiber	Fat	Protein	Score
0	0	12	0	F+

Tartar Sauce

What to gather

⅔ cup	Saffola Mayonnaise
2 spears	Kosher dill pickles, finely chopped
1 tbsp	Lime juice

Tartar Sauce

How to prepare

In small bowl, mix all ingredients until well combined. Serve chilled.

Nutrition Facts per Serving (approx 1 tbsp)

Usable Carbs	Fiber	Fat	Protein	Score
0	0	6	0	F+

Desserts

Pie Crust

What to gather

1½ cup	Hazelnut meal
¼ cup	Splenda for baking
2 tbsp	Butter, chilled
2 tbsp	Heavy whipping cream

How to prepare

In a food processor, blend all ingredients until dough is combined and clumps together. Chill for 15 minutes. Press pie dough into an 8″ nonstick pie pan and bake at 325° for 10 minutes.

Use with coconut cream pie recipe, page 332.

Almond Butter Cookies

What to gather

1 cup	Almond meal
¼ cup	Splenda for baking
2 tbsp	Butter, chilled
1½ tbsp	Heavy whipping cream
1	Egg
1 tsp	Almond extract
12	Almonds, whole

prep: moderate

How to prepare

In a food processor, blend all ingredients until dough clumps together. Chill for 15 minutes. Preheat oven to 350° F while cookie dough chills.

Using a tablespoon to measure out each cookie, roll dough into a ball and place on nonstick cookie sheet. Press a whole almond into the center of cookie. Repeat to create 11 more cookies with remaining dough.

Bake for 12-15 minutes or until golden brown.

Nutrition Facts per Serving

Usable Carbs	Fiber	Fat	Protein	Score
1	1	9	3	F+

Brownies

What to gather

1 cup	Torani sugar-free chocolate syrup
2 tbsp	Butter, salted
4 tbsp	Almond oil
4	Eggs
¼ cup	Flaxseed meal
¾ cup	Hazelnut meal
½ cup	Cocoa powder, unsweetened
¼ tsp	Baking powder
1 tsp	Vanilla extract
	Salt

How to prepare

Reduce chocolate syrup to ¼ cup.

Mix cooled chocolate syrup, butter, almond oil and eggs together. Add flax meal, hazelnut meal, cocoa powder, baking powder and a pinch of salt; mix well with a whisk. Stir in pure vanilla extract.

Pour into a buttered 6" square glass pan and bake at 325° F for 25-30 minutes or until an inserted toothpick comes out clean.

Nutrition Facts per Serving

Usable Carbs	Fiber	Fat	Protein	Score
2	4	19	6	F+

Coconut Cream Pie

What to gather

¼ cup	Coconut flakes, unsweetened
1½ cups	Torani sugar-free coconut syrup
½ tsp	Salt
2½ cups	Carb Countdown 2% milk
2 tbsp	Butter
2	Egg yolks
1 tsp	Vanilla extract
2 tsp	Coconut extract
¼ tsp	Xanthan gum (optional)
1½ cups	GNC PM Protein, vanilla caramel flavor
1	Pie crust, prepared page 326

Coconut Cream Pie

prep: involved

How to prepare

Reduce coconut syrup to ¾ cup. Let cool

Preheat oven to 350° F.

Bake coconut in a shallow pan 5 to 6 minutes or until toasted. Set aside.

Combine coconut syrup, salt and Carb Countdown 2% milk in a heavy saucepan. Cook over medium-high heat, whisking occasionally; bring to a boil. Remove from heat. Whisk in butter. In a separate bowl, whisk egg yolks until thick and pale. Gradually whisk ¾ cup of hot custard mixture into yolks; add to remaining hot custard mixture, whisking constantly. Add vanilla and coconut extracts, toasted coconut flakes, and xanthan gum (optional). Whisk in protein powder until thoroughly combined and custard begins to thicken, about 5-7 minutes. Pour filling into prepared piecrust. Cover with plastic wrap and chill 3 hours or until firm.

Nutrition Facts per Serving

Usable Carbs	Fiber	Fat	Protein	Score
4	3	25	11	F+

Creamy Cheese Gelato with Pecans

What to gather

1¼ cup   Parmesan cheese, finely grated

1½ cup   Heavy whipping cream

¼ tsp   White stevia powder

½ cup   Torani sugar-free caramel syrup

½ cup   Pecans, toasted

Creamy Cheese Gelato with Pecans

prep: involved

How to prepare

In a medium bowl add grated Parmesan cheese, heavy whipping cream and white stevia powder. Set over a medium pot of simmering water over medium-low heat. Whisk constantly until slightly thickened, 15-20 minutes. Strain into a wide 2-cup glass dish, cover, and refrigerate overnight.

Reduce caramel syrup to ¼ cup. Let cool.

To serve, put a scoop of cheese gelato on plate and top with warm syrup and toasted pecans.

Nutrition Facts per Serving

Usable Carbs	Fiber	Fat	Protein	Score
1	1	22	5	F+

Hazelnut Cookies

What to gather

1 cup	Hazelnut meal
¼ cup	Splenda for baking
2 tbsp	Butter, chilled
1½ tbsp	Heavy whipping cream
1	Egg
1 tsp	Vanilla extract

How to prepare

In a food processor, blend all ingredients until dough clumps together. Chill for 15 minutes. Preheat oven to 350° F while cookie dough chills.

Using a tablespoon to measure out each cookie, roll dough into a ball and place on nonstick cookie sheet. Press a whole almond into the center of cookie. Repeat to create 11 more cookies with remaining dough.

Bake for 12-15 minutes or until golden brown.

Nutrition Facts per Serving

Usable Carbs	Fiber	Fat	Protein	Score
2	2	12	3	F+

Hazelnut Iced Cream

What to gather

¾ cup	Heavy whipping cream
1¼ cups	Carb Countdown skim milk
1¼ scoops	GNC PM Protein, vanilla caramel flavor
¼ cup	Torani sugar-free hazelnut syrup

prep: basic

How to prepare

In a medium sized mixing bowl, whisk all ingredients until smooth. Pour mixture in a freezer-safe bowl and freeze for at least 5 hours. Remove iced cream from freezer and let stand at room temperature for 15-20 minutes to soften before serving.

Nutrition Facts per Serving

Usable Carbs	Fiber	Fat	Protein	Score
0	0	7	4	F

Beverages

Fat Irish Coffee

What to gather

1 cup	Coffee, prepared
2 tbsp	Heavy whipping cream
3 tbsp	Torani sugar-free Irish cream syrup
2 tbsp	Benefiber fiber supplement

prep: basic

How to prepare

In coffee cup, combine hot coffee (regular or decaf) and remaining ingredients with spoon. Stir intermittently while drinking.

Nutrition Facts per Serving

Usable Carbs	Fiber	Fat	Protein	Score
0	6	12	0	F+

Fruitless Fiber Smoothie

What to gather

1 scoop	No-carb protein powder
1 tbsp	Canola or flaxseed oil
1 tbsp	Colon Cleanse psyllium fiber
8-12 fl oz	Water

Fruitless Fiber Smoothie

prep: basic

How to prepare

Combine ingredients in large glass. Stir immediately and drink.

For extra-smooth and creamy texture

In blender, combine ingredients and blend for 30 seconds on high.

Nutrition Facts per Serving

Usable Carbs	Fiber	Fat	Protein	Score
1	5	14	20	N

Iced Mocha Latte

What to gather

½ cup	Torani sugar-free chocolate syrup
2 tbsp	Cocoa powder, unsweetened
2 tbsp	Instant coffee granules
2 cups	Boiling water
½ cup	Heavy whipping cream
1 cup	Carb Countdown chocolate milk

Iced Mocha Latte

How to prepare

In a small bowl, combine syrup, cocoa and coffee. Gradually whisk in boiling water; continue whisking until blended. Stir in whipping cream. Pour mixture into ice cube trays. Freeze for 8 hours.

Pour chocolate milk in blender. Gradually add frozen mocha cubes, blending on medium speed until smooth. Serve immediately.

Nutrition Facts per Serving

Usable Carbs	Fiber	Fat	Protein	Score
3	1	14	4	F+

Quinine Cooler

What to gather

8 oz	Diet Snapple Iced Tea, raspberry
6 oz	Diet tonic water
¼ cup	Torani sugar-free raspberry syrup

prep: basic

How to prepare

In large glass, combine all ingredients. Stir gently until mixed.
Serve chilled.

Other syrup and tea flavors may be used.

Nutrition Facts per Serving

Usable Carbs	Fiber	Fat	Protein	Score
0	0	0	0	N

Citations

Beginning The Journey

A

1. Meigs JB, D'Agostino RB Sr, Wilson PW, et al. Diabetes. 1997; 46: 1594-600.

2. Reaven GM. Diabetes. 1988; 37: 1595-607.

B

1. Dansinger ML, Gleason JA, Griffith JL, et al. JAMA. 2005; 293: 43-53.

C

1. Albu JB, Murphy L, Frager DH, et al. Diabetes. 1997; 46: 456-62.

2. Ascaso JF, Romero P, Real JT, et al. Eur J Intern Med. 2003; 14: 101-106.

3. Bigaard J, Tjonneland A, Thomsen BL, et al. Obes Res. 2003; 11: 895-903.

4. Booth ML, Hunter C, Gore CJ, et al. Int J Obes Relat Metab Disord. 2000; 24: 1058-61.

5. Caprio S, Hyman LD, Limb C, et al. Am J Physiol. 1995; 269(1 Pt 1): E118-26.

6. Carey DG, Jenkins AB, Campbell LV, et al. Diabetes. 1996; 45: 633-8.

7. Colman E, Toth MJ, Katzel LI, et al. Int J Obes Relat Metab Disord. 1995; 19: 798-803.

8. Coon PJ, Rogus EM, Drinkwater D, et al. J Clin Endocrinol Metab. 1992; 75: 1125-32.

9. Cornier MA, Tate CW, Grunwald GK, et al. Obes Res. 2002; 10: 1167-72.

10. Despres JP, Couillard C, Gagnon J, et al. Arterioscler Thromb Vasc Biol. 2000; 20: 1932-8.

11. DiPietro L, Katz LD, Nadel ER. Int J Obes Relat Metab Disord. 1999; 23: 432-6.

12. Freedman DS, Srinivasan SR, Burke GL, et al. Am J Clin Nutr. 1987; 46: 403-10.

13. Fujioka S, Matsuzawa Y, Tokunaga K, et al. Int J Obes. 1991; 15: 853-9.

14. Gabriely I, Ma XH, Yang XM, et al. Diabetes. 2002; 51: 2951-8.

15. Goodpaster BH, Krishnaswami S, Resnick H, et al. Diabetes Care. 2003; 26: 372-9.

16. Goulding A, Taylor RW, Jones IE, et al. Int J Obes Relat Metab Disord. 2000; 24: 627-32.

17. Harris MM, Stevens J, Thomas N, et al. Obes Res. 2000; 8: 516-24.

18. He Q, Horlick M, Fedun B, et al. Circulation. 2002; 105: 1093-8.

19. Hu D, Hannah J, Gray RS, et al. Obes Res. 2000; 8: 411-21.

20. Iwao S, Iwao N, Muller DC, et al. J Am Geriatr Soc. 2000; 48: 788-94.

21. Janssen I, Katzmarzyk PT, Ross R. Am J Clin Nutr. 2004; 79: 379-84.

22. Janssen I, Katzmarzyk PT, Ross R, et al. Obes Res. 2004; 12: 525-37.

23. Kim JY, Nolte LA, Hansen PA, et al. Am J Physiol Regul Integr Comp Physiol. 2000; 279: R2057-65.

24. Kriketos AD, Carey DG, Jenkins AB, et al. Diabet Med. 2003; 20: 294-300.

25. Krotkiewski M, Bjorntorp P, Sjostrom L, et al. J Clin Invest. 1983; 72: 1150-62.

26. Kunesova M, Hainer V, Hergetova H, et al. Sb Lek. 1995; 96: 257-67.

27. Kuo CS, Hwu CM, Chiang SC, et al. Diabetes Nutr Metab. 2002; 15: 101-8.

28. Laaksonen DE, Kainulainen S, Rissanen A, et al. Nutr Metab Cardiovasc Dis. 2003; 13: 349-56.

29. Lemieux S, Prud'homme D, Moorjani S, et al. Atherosclerosis. 1995; 118: 155-64.

30. Nestel PJ, Clifton PM, Noakes M, et al. J Hypertens. 1993; 11: 1387-94.

31. Nguyen-Duy TB, Nichaman MZ, Church TS, et al. Am J Physiol Endocrinol Metab. 2003; 284: E1065-71.

32. Nieves DJ, Cnop M, Retzlaff B, et al. Diabetes. 2003; 52: 172-9.

33. Obisesan TO, Toth MJ, Ades PA, et al. Exp Gerontol. 1997; 32: 643-51.

34. Odamaki M, Furuya R, Ohkawa S, et al. Nephrol Dial Transplant. 1999; 14: 2427-32.

35. Okosun IS, Cooper RS, Prewitt TE, et al. Ethn Dis. 1999; 9: 218-29.

The Carb Nite Solution

36. Okosun IS, Liao Y, Rotimi CN, et al. Ann Epidemiol. 2000; 10: 263-70.

37. Ouyang P, Sung J, Kelemen MD, et al. J Womens Health (Larchmt). 2004; 13: 177-85.

38. Pare A, Dumont M, Lemieux I, et al. Obes Res. 2001; 9: 526-34.

39. Pouliot MC, Despres JP, Lemieux S, et al. Am J Cardiol. 1994; 73: 460-8.

40. Rexrode KM, Buring JE, Manson JE. Int J Obes Relat Metab Disord. 2001; 25: 1047-56.

41. Ronnemaa T, Koskenvuo M, Marniemi J, et al. J Clin Endocrinol Metab. 1997; 82: 383-7.

42. Ronnemaa T, Marniemi J, Savolainen MJ, et al. J Clin Endocrinol Metab. 1998; 83: 2792-9.

43. Rosenfalck AM, Almdal T, Gotfredsen A, et al. Int J Obes Relat Metab Disord. 1996; 20: 1006-13.

44. Ross R, Katzmarzyk PT. Int J Obes Relat Metab Disord. 2003; 27: 204-10.

45. Ross SJ, Poehlman ET, Johnson RK, et al. J Cardiopulm Rehabil. 1997; 17: 419-27.

46. Sardinha LB, Teixeira PJ, Guedes DP, et al. Metabolism. 2000; 49: 1379-85.

47. Seidell JC, Perusse L, Despres JP, et al. Am J Clin Nutr. 2001; 74: 315-21.

48. Svendsen OL, Hassager C, Christiansen C. Int J Obes Relat Metab Disord. 1993; 17: 459-63.

49. T S Han, E M van Leer, J C Seidell, et al. BMJ. 1995; 311: 1401-1405.

50. Tchernof A, Lamarche B, Prud'Homme D, et al. Diabetes Care. 1996; 19: 629-37.

51. Van Pelt RE, Evans EM, Schechtman KB, et al. Am J Physiol Endocrinol Metab. 2002; 282: E1023-8.

52. Weyer C, Foley JE, Bogardus C, et al. Diabetologia. 2000; 43: 1498-506.

53. Williams MJ, Hunter GR, Kekes-Szabo T, et al. Am J Clin Nutr. 1997; 65: 855-60.

54. Wong SL, Katzmarzyk P, Nichaman MZ, et al. Med Sci Sports Exerc. 2004; 36: 286-91.

55. Yagalla MV, Hoerr SL, Song WO, et al. J Am Diet Assoc. 1996; 96: 257-61.

56. Zhao LC, Wu YF, Li Y, et al. Zhonghua Yu Fang Yi Xue Za Zhi. 2003; 37: 346-50.

57. Zhao LC, Wu YF, Zhou BF, et al. Zhonghua Liu Xing Bing Xue Za Zhi. 2003; 24: 471-5.

58. Zhu S, Wang Z, Heshka S, et al. Am J Clin Nutr. 2002; 76: 743-9.

Often Ignored Hazards

A

1. Allison DB, Zannolli R, Faith MS, Heo M, Pietrobelli A, Vanitallie TB, Pi-Sunyer FX, Heymsfield SB. Weight loss increases and fat loss decreaess all-cause mortality rate: results from two independent cohort studies. Presented at: ACSM 46th Annual meeting, 1999.

2. Atkinson RL. Ann Intern Med. 1993; 119(7 Pt 2): 677-80.

3. Bakker I, Twisk JW, Van Mechelen W, et al. J Clin Endocrinol Metab. 2003; 88: 2607-13.

4. Behrens L, Kerschensteiner M, Misgeld T, et al. J Immunol. 1998; 164: 5330.

5. Chan MH, Carey AL, Watt MJ, et al. Am J Physiol Regul Integr Comp Physiol. 2004; 287: R322-7.

6. Cicoira M, Davos CH, Francis DP, et al. J Card Fail. 2004; 10: 421-6.

7. Croisier JL, Camus G, Venneman I, et al. Muscle Nerve. 1999; 22: 208-12.

8. Goebels N, Michaelis D, Wekerle H, et al. J Immunol. 1992; 149: 661-7.

9. Hiscock N, Chan MH, Bisucci T, et al. FASEB J. 2004; 18: 992-4.

10. Hohlfeld R, Engel AG. Immunol Today. 1994; 15: 269-74.

11. Jonsdottir IH, Schjerling P, Ostrowski K, et al. J Physiol. 2000; 528 Pt 1: 157-63.

12. Keller C, Steensberg A, Pilegaard H, et al. FASEB J. 2001; 15: 2748-50.

13. Keller P, Keller C, Carey AL, et al. Biochem Biophys Res Commun. 2003; 310: 550-4.

14. MacDonald C, Wojtaszewski JF, Pedersen BK, et al. J Appl Physiol. 2003; 95: 2273-7.

15. Nagaraju K, Raben N, Villalba ML, et al. Clin Immunol. 1999; 92: 161-9.

16. Nieman DC, Nehlsen-Cannarella SI, Henson DA, et al. Int J Obes Relat Metab Disord. 1996; 20: 353-60.

17. Okura T, Nakata Y, Yamabuki K, et al. Arterioscler Thromb Vasc Biol. 2004; 24: 923-9.

18. Ostrowski K, Rohde T, Zacho M, et al. J Physiol. 1998; 508 (Pt 3): 949-53.

19. Pedersen BK, Steensberg A, Fischer C, et al. Exerc Immunol Rev. 2001; 7: 18-31.

20. Starkie RL, Arkinstall MJ, Koukoulas I, et al. J Physiol. 2001; 533(Pt 2): 585-91.

21. Steensberg A, Febbraio MA, Osada T, et al. J Physiol. 2001; 537(Pt 2): 633-9.

22. Steensberg A, Keller C, Starkie RL, et al. Am J Physiol Endocrinol Metab. 2002; 283: E1272-8.

23. Steensberg A, van Hall G, Osada T, et al. J Physiol. 2000; 529 Pt 1: 237-42.

24. Wiendl H, Mitsdoerffer M, Schneider D, et al. FASEB J. 2003; 17: 1892-4.

25. Wiendl H, Mitsdoerffer M, Schneider D, et al. Brain. 2003; 126(Pt 5): 1026-35.

B

1. Doucet E, Tremblay A, Simoneau JA, et al. Am J Clin Nutr. 2003; 78: 430-5.

2. Dulloo AG, Jacquet J, Girardier L. Int J Obes Relat Metab Disord. 1996; 20: 393-405.

3. Heshka S, Yang MU, Wang J, et al. Am J Clin Nutr. 1990; 52: 981-6.

4. Kreitzman SN, Coxon AY, Johnson PG, et al. Am J Clin Nutr. 1992; 56(1 Suppl): 258S-261S.

5. Layman DK. J Nutr. 2003; 133: 261S-267S.

6. Schwingshandl J, Borkenstein M. Int J Obes Relat Metab Disord. 1995; 19: 752-5.

7. Sergi G, Coin A, Bussolotto M, et al. J Gerontol A Biol Sci Med Sci. 2002; 57: M302-7.

8. Sheu WH, Chin HM, Su HY, et al. Clin Exp Hypertens. 1998; 20: 403-16.

9. Toubro S, Christensen NJ, Astrup A. Int J Obes Relat Metab Disord. 1995; 19: 544-9.

10. Verga S, Buscemi S, Vaccaro M, et al. Recenti Prog Med. 1989; 80: 574-6.

11. Wang Z, Heshka S, Gallagher D, et al. Am J Physiol Endocrinol Metab. 2000; 279: E539-45.

12. Zhang K, Sun M, Werner P, et al. Int J Obes Relat Metab Disord. 2002; 26: 376-83.

C

1. Barzilai N, Gupta G. J Gerontol A Biol Sci Med Sci. 1999; 54: B89-96; discussion B97-8.

2. Dhar HL. Indian J Med Sci. 1999; 53: 390-2.

3. Hansen BC. J Nutr. 2001; 131: 900S-902S.

4. Hansen BC, Bodkin NL, Ortmeyer HK. Toxicol Sci. 1999; 52(2 Suppl): 56-60.

5. Heilbronn LK, Ravussin E. Am J Clin Nutr. 2003; 78: 361-9.

6. Ingram DK, Anson RM, de Cabo R, et al. Ann N Y Acad Sci. 2004; 1019: 412-23.

7. Lane MA, Ingram DK, Roth GS. Toxicol Sci. 1999; 52(2 Suppl): 41-8.

8. Lane MA, Tilmont EM, De Angelis H, et al. Mech Ageing Dev. 2000; 112: 185-96.

9. Spindler SR. Ann N Y Acad Sci. 2001; 928: 296-304.

10. Toussaint O, Remacle J, Dierick JF, et al. Mech Ageing Dev. 2002; 123: 937-46.

D

1. Bjorntorp P, Sjostrom L. Adipose tissue dysfunction and its consequences. In: New Perspectives in Adipose Tissue Development: Structure, Function, and Development, edited by A. Cryer, and R. L. R. Van. London: Butterworths, 1985, p. 447-485.

2. Brook CG, Lloyd JK, Wolf OH. Br Med J. 1972; 2: 25-7.

3. Choi YH, Li CL, Hartzell DL, et al. Domest Anim Endocrinol. 2003; 25: 295-301.

4. Commins SP, Watson PM, Frampton IC, et al. Am J Physiol Endocrinol Metab. 2001; 280: E372-7.

5. Deslex S, Negrel R, Vannier C, et al. Int J Obes. 1987; 11: 19-27.

6. Faust IM, Johnson PR, Stern JS, et al. Am J Physiol Endocrinol Metab. 1978; 235: E279-E286.

7. Faust IM, Miller WH Jr, Sclafani A, et al. Am J Physiol. 1984; 247(6 Pt 2): R1038-46.

8. Gregoire FM, Smas CM, Sul HS. Physiol Rev. 1998; 78: 783-809.

9. Gullicksen PS, Hausman DB, Dean RG, et al. Int J Obes Relat Metab Disord. 2003; 27: 302-12.

10. Johnson PR, Stern JS, Greenwood MRC, et al. Metab. 1978; 27(Suppl 2): 1941-1954.

11. Kras KM, Hausman DB, Martin RJ. Obes Res. 2000; 8: 186-93.

12. Lau DC, Shillabeer G, Wong KL, et al. Int J Obes. 1990; 14 Suppl 3: 193-201.

13. Lau DCW, Shillabeer G, Li Z-H, et al. Int J Obes. 1996; 20: S16-S25.

14. Loftus TM, Kuhajda FP, Lane MD. Proc Natl Acad Sci U S A. 1998; 95: 14168-72.

15. Marques BG, Hausman DB, Martin RJ. Am J Physiol. 1998; 275(6 Pt 2): R1898-908.

16. Miller WH Jr, Faust IM, Hirsch J. J Lipid Res. 1984; 25: 336-47.

17. Prins JB, Niesler CU, Winterford CM, et al. Diabetes. 1997; 46: 1939-44.

18. Prins JB, O'Rahilly S. Clin Sci (Lond). 1997; 92: 3-11.

19. Prins JB, Walker NI, Winterford CM, et al. Biochem Biophys Res Commun. 1994; 201: 500-7.

20. Qian H, Azain MJ, Compton MM, et al. Endocrinology. 1998; 139: 791-4.

21. Serrero G, Lepak N. Obesity. 1996; 20: S58-S64.

E

1. Abate N, Haffner SM, Garg A, et al. J Clin Endocrinol Metab. 2002; 87: 4522-7.

2. Andersson B, Marin P, Lissner L, et al. Diabetes Care. 1994; 17: 405-11.

3. Arner P, Bolinder J, Engfeldt P, et al. Metabolism. 1981; 30: 753-60.

4. Astrup A, Grunwald GK, Melanson EL, et al. Int J Obes Relat Metab Disord. 2000; 24: 1545-52.

5. Astrup A, Ryan L, Grunwald GK, et al. Br J Nutr. 2000; 83 Suppl 1: S25-32.

6. Backberg M, Hervieu G, Wilson S, et al. Eur J Neurosci. 2002; 15: 315-28.

7. Baghaei F, Rosmond R, Westberg L, et al. Obes Res. 2003; 11: 578-85.

8. Barba G, Russo O, Siani A, et al. Obes Res. 2003; 11: 160-6.

9. Baskin DG, Breininger JF, Schwartz MW. Diabetes. 1999; 48: 828-33.

10. Baskin DG, Seeley RJ, Kuijper JL, et al. Diabetes. 1998; 47: 538-43.

11. Bellone S, Rapa A, Vivenza D, et al. J Endocrinol Invest. 2002; 25: RC13-5.

12. Bernasconi D, Del Monte P, Meozzi M, et al. Metabolism. 1996; 45: 72-5.

13. Brunner L, Nick HP, Cumin F, et al. Int J Obes Relat Metab Disord. 1997; 21: 1152-60.

14. Buscemi S, Verga S, Maneri R, et al. A 3-3. 1997; 20: 276-81.

15. Campfield LA, Smith FJ, Burn P. Horm Metab Res. 1996; 28: 619-32.

16. Campfield LA, Smith FJ, Guisez Y, et al. Science. 1995; 269: 546-9.

17. Chan JL, Bullen J, Lee JH, et al. J Clin Endocrinol Metab. 2004; 89: 335-43.

18. Cheung CC, Clifton DK, Steiner RA. Endocrinology. 1997; 138: 4489-92.

19. Chomard P, Beltramo JL, Ben Cheikh R, et al. J Endocrinol. 1994; 142: 317-24.

20. Chomard P, Vernhes G, Autissier N, et al. Hum Nutr Clin Nutr. 1985; 39: 371-8.

21. Cohen P, Zhao C, Cai X, et al. J Clin Invest. 2001; 108: 1113-21.

22. Considine RV, Sinha MK, Heiman ML, et al. N Engl J Med. 1996; 334: 292-5.

23. Cummings DE, Weigle DS, Frayo RS, et al. N Engl J Med. 2002; 346: 1623-30.

24. Daminet S, Jeusette I, Duchateau L, et al. J Vet Med A Physiol Pathol Clin Med. 2003; 50: 213-8.

25. De Pergola G, Triggiani V, Giorgino F, et al. Int J Obes Relat Metab Disord. 1994; 18: 659-64.

26. Di Marzo V, Goparaju SK, Wang L, et al. Nature. 2001; 410: 822-5.

27. Djuric Z, Lababidi S, Heilbrun LK, et al. J Am Coll Nutr. 2002; 21: 38-46.

28. Douyon L, Schteingart DE. Endocrinol Metab Clin North Am. 2002; 31: 173-89.

29. Drago F, Lo Presti L, Nardo F, et al. Biol Reprod. 1982; 27: 765-70.

30. Dryden S, King P, Pickavance L, et al. Clin Sci (Lond). 1999; 96: 307-12.

31. Duntas L, Hauner H, Rosenthal J, et al. Int J Obes. 1991; 15: 83-7.

32. Elbers JM, Asscheman H, Seidell JC, et al. J Clin Endocrinol Metab. 1997; 82: 2044-7.

33. Elias CF, Lee C, Kelly J, et al. Neuron. 1998; 21: 1375-85.

34. Elmquist JK. Physiol Behav. 2001; 74(4-5): 703-8.

35. Ersoz H, Onde ME, Terekeci H, et al. Int J Androl. 2002; 25: 312-6.

36. Evans DJ, Hoffmann RG, Kalkhoff RK, et al. J Clin Endocrinol Metab. 1983; 57: 304-10.

37. Fagerberg B, Hulten LM, Hulthe J. Metabolism. 2003; 52: 1460-3.

38. Fisher JS, Hickner RC, Racette SB, et al. J Clin Endocrinol Metab. 1999; 84: 3726-31.

39. Fruhbeck G, Aguado M, Gomez-Ambrosi J, et al. Biochem Biophys Res Commun. 1998; 250: 99-102.

40. Fruhbeck G, Aguado M, Martinez JA. Biochem Biophys Res Commun. 1997; 240: 590-4.

41. Fruhbeck G, Gomez-Ambrosi J. Med Sci Monit. 2002; 8: BR47-55.

42. Fruhbeck G, Gomez-Ambrosi J, Salvador J. FASEB J. 2001; 15: 333-40.

43. Funahashi H, Hori T, Shimoda Y, et al. Regul Pept. 2000; 92(1-3): 31-5.

44. Gapstur SM, Gann PH, Kopp P, et al. Cancer Epidemiol Biomarkers Prev. 2002; 11(10 Pt 1): 1041-7.

45. Goldstone AP, Mercer JG, Gunn I, et al. FEBS Lett. 1997; 415: 134-8.

46. Groop LC, Bonadonna RC, Simonson DC, et al. Am J Physiol. 1992; 263(1 Pt 1): E79-84.

47. Haffner SM, Bauer RL. Int J Obes Relat Metab Disord. 1992; 16: 869-74.

48. Haffner SM, Katz MS, Dunn JF. Int J Obes. 1991; 15: 471-8.

49. Haffner SM, Valdez RA, Stern MP, et al. Int J Obes Relat Metab Disord. 1993; 17: 643-9.

50. Halaas JL, Gajiwala KS, Maffei M, et al. Science. 1995; 269: 543-6.

51. Hansen TK, Dall R, Hosoda H, et al. Clin Endocrinol (Oxf). 2002; 56: 203-6.

52. Hassink SG, Sheslow DV, de Lancey E, et al. Pediatrics. 1996; 98(2 Pt 1): 201-3.

53. Heini AF, Lara-Castro C, Kirk KA, et al. Int J Obes Relat Metab Disord. 1998; 22: 1084-7.

54. Hickey MS, Considine RV, Israel RG, et al. Am J Physiol. 1996; 271(5 Pt 1): E938-40.

55. Hosoi T, Okuma Y, Nomura Y. Biochem Biophys Res Commun. 2002; 294: 215-9.

56. Hosoi T, Okuma Y, Nomura Y. Brain Res. 2002; 949(1-2): 139-46.

57. Hube F, Lietz U, Igel M, et al. Horm Metab Res. 1996; 28: 690-3.

58. Ibanez L, Ong K, de Zegher F, et al. Clin Endocrinol (Oxf). 2003; 58: 372-9.

59. Ivandic A, Prpic-Krizevac I, Bozic D, et al. Wien Klin Wochenschr. 2002; 114(8-9): 321-6.

60. Ivandic A, Prpic-Krizevac I, Sucic M, et al. Metabolism. 1998; 47: 13-9.

61. Jankowska EA, Rogucka E, Medras M, et al. Med Sci Monit. 2000; 6: 1159-64.

62. Jequier E, Schutz Y. Am J Clin Nutr. 1983; 38: 989-98.

63. Kamohara S, Burcelin R, Halaas JL, et al. Nature. 1997; 389: 374-7.

64. Kaye SA, Folsom AR, Soler JT, et al. Int J Epidemiol. 1991; 20: 151-6.

65. Khaw KT, Barrett-Connor E. Ann Epidemiol. 1992; 2: 675-82.

66. Klein S, Coppack SW, Mohamed-Ali V, et al. Diabetes. 1996; 45: 984-7.

67. Kley HK, Deselaers T, Peerenboom H. Horm Metab Res. 1981; 13: 639-41.

68. Kley HK, Deselaers T, Peerenboom H, et al. J Clin Endocrinol Metab. 1980; 51: 1128-32.

69. Korner J, Savontaus E, Chua SC Jr, et al. J Neuroendocrinol. 2001; 13: 959-66.

70. Kristensen P, Judge ME, Thim L, et al. Nature. 1998; 393: 72-6.

71. Krotkiewski M, Kral JG, Karlsson J. Acta Physiol Scand. 1980; 109: 233-7.

72. Krsek M, Rosicka M, Papezova H, et al. Eat Weight Disord. 2003; 8: 207-11.

73. Kunesova M, Hainer V, Obenberger J, et al. Sb Lek. 2002; 103: 477-85.

74. Kvetny J. Horm Res. 1985; 21: 60-5.

75. Lala VR, Ray A, Jamias P, et al. J Am Coll Nutr. 1988; 7: 361-6.

76. Lederer J. (author's transl). 1980; 56(29-32): 1237-40.

77. Leenen R, van der Kooy K, Seidell JC, et al. J Clin Endocrinol Metab. 1994; 78: 1515-20.

78. Lindeman JH, Pijl H, Van Dielen FM, et al. Obes Res. 2002; 10: 1161-6.

79. Longcope C, Pratt JH, Schneider SH, et al. J Clin Endocrinol Metab. 1978; 46: 146-52.

80. Lonnqvist F, Nordfors L, Jansson M, et al. J Clin Invest. 1997; 99: 2398-404.

81. Lukanova A, Lundin E, Zeleniuch-Jacquotte A, et al. Eur J Endocrinol. 2004; 150: 161-71.

82. Malik IA, English PJ, Ghatei MA, et al. Clin Endocrinol (Oxf). 2004; 60: 137-41.

83. Mantzoros CS, Georgiadis EI, Evangelopoulou K, et al. Epidemiology. 1996; 7: 513-6.

84. Marzullo P, Verti B, Savia G, et al. J Clin Endocrinol Metab. 2004; 89: 936-9.

85. Matzen LE, Kvetny J, Pedersen KK. Scand J Clin Lab Invest. 1989; 49: 249-53.

86. Mercer JG, Hoggard N, Williams LM, et al. J Neuroendocrinol. 1996; 8: 733-5.

87. Mercer JG, Moar KM, Rayner DV, et al. FEBS Lett. 1997; 402(2-3): 185-8.

88. Minocci A, Savia G, Lucantoni R, et al. Int J Obes Relat Metab Disord. 2000; 24: 1139-44.

89. Mistry AM, Swick AG, Romsos DR. J Nutr. 1997; 127: 2065-72.

90. Moberg E, Sjoberg S, Hagstrom-Toft E, et al. Am J Physiol Endocrinol Metab. 2002; 283: E295-301.

91. Moinat M, Deng C, Muzzin P, et al. FEBS Lett. 1995; 373: 131-4.

92. Moller N, O'Brien P, Nair KS. J Clin Endocrinol Metab. 1998; 83: 931-4.

93. Morley JE, Alshaher MM, Farr SA, et al. Peptides. 1999; 20: 595-600.

94. Mueller-Cunningham WM, Quintana R, Kasim-Karakas SE. J Am Diet Assoc. 2003; 103: 1600-6.

95. Nedeljkovic B, Kmezic-Slavic V, Sekulic J. Med Pregl. 1993; 46(1-2): 11-4.

96. Niimi M, Sato M, Taminato T. Endocrine. 2001; 14: 269-73.

97. Ostlund RE Jr, Yang JW, Klein S, et al. J Clin Endocrinol Metab. 1996; 81: 3909-13.

98. Otto B, Cuntz U, Fruehauf E, et al. Eur J Endocrinol. 2001; 145: 669-73.

99. Pelleymounter MA, Cullen MJ, Baker MB, et al. Science. 1995; 269: 540-3.

100. Pinto S, Roseberry AG, Liu H, et al. Science. 2004; 304: 110-5.

101. Proulx K, Richard D, Walker CD. Endocrinology. 2002; 143: 4683-92.

102. Raben A, Jensen ND, Marckmann P, et al. Int J Obes Relat Metab Disord. 1995; 19: 916-23.

103. Ramsay TG. J Anim Sci. 2001; 79: 653-7.

104. Reinehr T, Andler W. Arch Dis Child. 2002; 87: 320-3.

105. Rentsch J, Levens N, Chiesi M. Biochem Biophys Res Commun. 1995; 214: 131-6.

106. Rigamonti AE, Pincelli AI, Corra B, et al. J Endocrinol. 2002; 175: R1-5.

107. Rock CL, Thomson C, Caan BJ, et al. Cancer. 2001; 91: 25-34.

108. Ronnemaa T, Karonen SL, Rissanen A, et al. Ann Intern Med. 1997; 126: 26-31.

109. Rosicka M, Krsek M, Matoulek M, et al. Physiol Res. 2003; 52: 61-6.

110. Roti E, Minelli R, Salvi M. Int J Obes Relat Metab Disord. 2000; 24 Suppl 2: S113-5.

111. Sahu A. Endocrinology. 1998; 139: 795-8.

112. Sari R, Balci MK, Altunbas H, et al. Clin Endocrinol (Oxf). 2003; 59: 258-62.

113. Schwartz MW, Baskin DG, Bukowski TR, et al. Diabetes. 1996; 45: 531-5.

114. Schwartz MW, Erickson JC, Baskin DG, et al. Endocrinology. 1998; 139: 2629-35.

115. Schwartz MW, Seeley RJ, Campfield LA, et al. J Clin Invest. 1996; 98: 1101-6.

116. Seidell JC, Cigolini M, Charzewska J, et al. J Clin Epidemiol. 1990; 43: 21-34.

117. Shimada M, Tritos NA, Lowell BB, et al. Nature. 1998; 396: 670-4.

118. Shimizu H, Shimomura Y, Hayashi R, et al. Int J Obes Relat Metab Disord. 1997; 21: 536-41.

119. Siegrist-Kaiser CA, Pauli V, Juge-Aubry CE, et al. J Clin Invest. 1997; 100: 2858-64.

120. Skov AR, Toubro S, Buemann B, et al. Clin Physiol. 1997; 17: 279-85.

121. Soderberg S, Olsson T, Eliasson M, et al. Int J Obes Relat Metab Disord. 2001; 25: 98-105.

122. Soriano-Guillen L, Barrios V, Campos-Barros A, et al. J Pediatr. 2004; 144: 36-42.

123. Soukup T, Zacharova G, Smerdu V, et al. Physiol Res. 2001; 50: 619-26.

124. Stephens TW, Basinski M, Bristow PK, et al. Nature. 1995; 377: 530-2.

125. Stichel H, l'Allemand D, Gruters A. Horm Res. 2000; 54: 14-9.

126. Stokholm KH, Lindgreen P. Int J Obes. 1982; 6: 573-8.

127. Stoney RM, Walker KZ, Bost JD, et al. Diabetes Care. 1998; 21: 828-30.

128. Strata A, Ugolotti G, Contini C, et al. Int J Obes. 1978; 2: 333-40.

129. Svendsen OL, Hassager C, Christiansen C. Int J Obes Relat Metab Disord. 1993; 17: 459-63.

130. Tagliaferri M, Berselli ME, Calo G, et al. Obes Res. 2001; 9: 196-201.

131. Tanaka M, Naruo T, Muranaga T, et al. Eur J Endocrinol. 2002; 146: R1-3.

132. Tassone F, Broglio F, Destefanis S, et al. J Clin Endocrinol Metab. 2003; 88: 5478-83.

133. Taylor RW, Goulding A. Aust N Z J Med. 1998; 28: 316-21.

134. Tsai EC, Matsumoto AM, Fujimoto WY, et al. Diabetes Care. 2004; 27: 861-8.

135. Tschop M, Weyer C, Tataranni PA, et al. Diabetes. 2001; 50: 707-9.

136. Van Den Saffele JK, Goemaere S, De Bacquer D, et al. Clin Endocrinol (Oxf). 1999; 51: 81-8.

137. Van Harmelen V, Reynisdottir S, Eriksson P, et al. Diabetes. 1998; 47: 913-7.

138. Wang MY, Lee Y, Unger RH. J Biol Chem. 1999; 274: 17541-4.

139. Wang ZW, Zhou YT, Lee Y, et al. Biochem Biophys Res Commun. 1999; 260: 653-7.

140. Wauters M, Mertens I, Considine R, et al. Eat Weight Disord. 1998; 3: 124-30.

141. William WN Jr, Ceddia RB, Curi R. J Endocrinol. 2002; 175: 735-44.

142. Winters SJ, Brufsky A, Weissfeld J, et al. Metabolism. 2001; 50: 1242-7.

143. Woodhouse LJ, Gupta N, Bhasin M, et al. J Clin Endocrinol Metab. 2004; 89: 718-26.

144. Zumoff B, Strain GW, Miller LK, et al. J Clin Endocrinol Metab. 1990; 71: 929-31.

F

1. Adami S, Ferrari M, Galvanini G, et al. J Endocrinol Invest. 1979; 2: 271-4.

2. Anderson IM, Crook WS, Gartside SE, et al. J Affect Disord. 1989; 16(2-3): 197-202.

3. Badger TM, Lynch EA, Fox PH. J Nutr. 1985; 115: 788-97.

4. Barrows K, Snook JT. Am J Clin Nutr. 1987; 45: 391-8.

5. Bates GW, Whitworth NS. Fertil Steril. 1982; 38: 406-9.

6. Beitins IZ, Barkan A, Klibanski A, et al. J Clin Endocrinol Metab. 1985; 60: 1120-6.

7. Bergendahl M, Vance ML, Iranmanesh A, et al. J Clin Endocrinol Metab. 1996; 81: 692-9.

8. Boden G, Chen X, Mozzoli M, et al. J Clin Endocrinol Metab. 1996; 81: 3419-3423.

9. Bryson JM, King SE, Burns CM, et al. Int J Obes Relat Metab Disord. 1996; 20: 338-45.

10. Burgess NS. J Am Diet Assoc. 1991; 91: 430-4.

11. Cameron JL, Weltzin TE, McConaha C, et al. J Clin Endocrinol Metab. 1991; 73: 35-41.

12. Carantoni M, Abbasi F, Azhar S, et al. J Clin Endocrinol Metab. 1999; 84: 869-72.

13. Cavallo E, Armellini F, Zamboni M, et al. Horm Metab Res. 1990; 22: 632-5.

14. Cella F, Adami GF, Giordano G, et al. Int J Obes Relat Metab Disord. 1999; 23: 494-7.

15. Challet E, le Maho Y, Robin JP, et al. Pharmacol Biochem Behav. 1995; 50: 405-12.

16. Chomard P, Vernhes G, Autissier N, et al. Eur J Clin Nutr. 1988; 42: 285-93.

17. Covasa M, Marcuson JK, Ritter RC. Am J Physiol Regul Integr Comp Physiol. 2001; 280: R331-7.

18. Cummings DE, Weigle DS, Frayo RS, et al. N Engl J Med. 2002; 346: 1623-30.

19. Davies HJ, Baird IM, Fowler J, et al. Am J Clin Nutr. 1989; 49: 745-51.

20. Doucet E, Pomerleau M, Harper ME. J Clin Endocrinol Metab. 2004; 89: 1727-32.

21. Doucet E, St Pierre S, Almeras N, et al. J Clin Endocrinol Metab. 2000; 85: 1550-6.

22. Dubuc GR, Phinney SD, Stern JS, et al. Metabolism. 1998; 47: 429–434.

23. Dulloo AG, Jacquet J. Am J Clin Nutr. 1998; 68: 599-606.

24. Escobar L, Freire JM, Giron JA, et al. Rev Esp Med Nucl. 2000; 19: 199-206.

25. French SJ, Murray B, Rumsey RD, et al. Br J Nutr. 1995; 73: 179-89.

26. Froidevaux F, Schutz Y, Christin L, et al. Am J Clin Nutr. 1993; 57: 35-42.

27. Garrel DR, Todd KS, Pugeat MM, et al. Am J Clin Nutr. 1984; 39: 930-6.

28. Geldszus R, Mayr B, Horn R, et al. Eur J Endocrinol. 1996; 135: 659-62.

29. Grant AM, Edwards OM, Howard AN, et al. Clin Endocrinol (Oxf). 1978; 9: 227-31.

30. Grinspoon SK, Askari H, Landt ML, et al. Am J Clin Nutr. 1997; 66: 1352–1356.

31. Guldstrand M, Backman L, Adamson U, et al. Diabetes Obes Metab. 1999; 1: 53-5.

32. Halle M, Berg A, Garwers U, et al. Am J Physiol. 1999; 277(2 Pt 1): E277-82.

33. Hansen TK, Dall R, Hosoda H, et al. Clin Endocrinol (Oxf). 2002; 56: 203-6.

34. Hanusch-Enserer U, Cauza E, Brabant G, et al. J Clin Endocrinol Metab. 2004; 89: 3352-8.

35. Hirschberg AL, Lindholm C, Carlstrom K, et al. Metabolism. 1994; 43: 217-22.

36. Hoffer LJ, Beitins IZ, Kyung NH, et al. J Clin Endocrinol Metab. 1986; 62: 288-92.

37. Hoffman RP, Stumbo PJ, Janz KF, et al. Horm Res. 1995; 44: 17-22.

38. Hramiak IM, Nisker JA. Am J Obstet Gynecol. 1985; 151: 264-7.

39. Infanger D, Baldinger R, Branson R, et al. Obes Surg. 2003; 13: 879-88.

40. Karklin A, Driver HS, Buffenstein R. Am J Clin Nutr. 1994; 59: 346-9.

41. Kather H, Scheurer A, Schlierf G. Int J Obes. 1987; 11: 191-200.

42. Kaukua J, Pekkarinen T, Sane T, et al. Obes Res. 2003; 11: 689-94.

43. Keim NL, Stern JS, Havel PJ. Am J Clin Nutr. 1998; 68: 794-801.

44. Kiddy DS, Hamilton-Fairley D, Seppala M, et al. Clin Endocrinol (Oxf). 1989; 31: 757-63.

45. Kiortsis DN, Durack I, Turpin G. Eur J Pediatr. 1999; 158: 446-50.

46. Klibanski A, Beitins IZ, Badger T, et al. J Clin Endocrinol Metab. 1981; 53: 258-63.

47. Krotkiewski M, Toss L, Bjorntorp P, et al. Int J Obes. 1981; 5: 287-93.

48. Krsek M, Rosicka M, Papezova H, et al. Eat Weight Disord. 2003; 8: 207-11.

49. Langendonk JG, Pijl H, Toornvliet AC, et al. J Clin Endocrinol Metab. 1998; 83: 1706-12.

50. Leenen R, van der Kooy K, Seidell JC, et al. J Clin Endocrinol Metab. 1994; 78: 1515-20.

51. Leidy HJ, Gardner JK, Frye BR, et al. J Clin Endocrinol Metab. 2004; 89: 2659-64.

52. Loucks AB, Heath EM. J Clin Endocrinol Metab. 1994; 78: 910-5.

53. Loucks AB, Verdun M, Heath EM. J Appl Physiol. 1998; 84: 37-46.

54. Luke A, Schoeller DA. Metabolism. 1992; 41: 450-6.

55. Marugo M, Bagnasco M, Contessini M, et al. J Endocrinol Invest. 1984; 7: 197-200.

56. Mathur R, Manchanda SK. Prog Neuropsychopharmacol Biol Psychiatry. 1991; 15: 405-13.

57. Matson CA, Ritter RC. Am J Physiol. 1999; 276(4 Pt 2): R1038-45.

58. Mavri A, Stegnar M, Sabovic M. Diabetes Obes Metab. 2001; 3: 293-6.

59. McLaughlin T, Abbasi F, Carantoni M, et al. J Clin Endocrinol Metab. 1999; 84: 578-81.

60. McMinn JE, Sindelar DK, Havel PJ, et al. Endocrinology. 2000; 141: 4442-8.

61. Menozzi R, Bondi M, Baldini A, et al. Br J Nutr. 2000; 84: 515-20.

62. Miyawaki T, Masuzaki H, Ogawa Y, et al. Eur J Clin Nutr. 2002; 56: 593-600.

63. Moinade S, Glanddier Y, Lambert M. Pathol Biol (Paris). 1985; 33: 27-33.

64. Moreira-Andres MN, Black EG, Ramsden DB, et al. Clin Endocrinol (Oxf). 1980; 12: 249-55.

65. Moreira-Andres MN, Del Canizo-Gomez FJ, Black EG, et al. Clin Endocrinol (Oxf). 1981; 15: 621-6.

66. Morpurgo PS, Resnik M, Agosti F, et al. J Endocrinol Invest. 2003; 26: 723-7.

67. Naslund E, Andersson I, Degerblad M, et al. J Intern Med. 2000; 248: 299-308.

68. Nelson KM, Weinsier RL. James LD. et al. Am J Clin Nutr. 1992; 55: 924-33.

69. Nicklas BJ, Katzel LI, Ryan AS, et al. Obes Res. 1997; 5: 62-8.

70. Niskanen L, Laaksonen DE, Punnonen K, et al. Diabetes Obes Metab. 2004; 6: 208-15.

71. O'Brian JT, Bybee DE, Burman KD, et al. Metabolism. 1980; 29: 721-7.

72. Osburne RC, Myers EA, Rodbard D, et al. Metabolism. 1983; 32: 9-13.

73. Pelletier C, Doucet E, Imbeault P, et al. Toxicol Sci. 2002; 67: 46-51.

74. Perreault M, Istrate N, Wang L, et al. Int J Obes Relat Metab Disord. 2004; 28: 879-85.

75. Rabast U, Hahn A, Reiners C, et al. Int J Obes. 1981; 5: 305-11.

76. Racette SB, Kohrt WM, Landt M, et al. Am J Clin Nutr. 1997; 66: 33-7.

77. Reiterer EE, Sudi KM, Mayer A, et al. J Pediatr Endocrinol Metab. 1999; 12: 853-62.

78. Romijn JA, Adriaanse R, Brabant G, et al. J Clin Endocrinol Metab. 1990; 70: 1631-6.

79. Samuels MH, Kramer P. J Clin Endocrinol Metab. 1996; 81: 32-6.

80. Samuels MH, McDaniel PA. J Clin Endocrinol Metab. 1997; 82: 3700-4.

81. Sari R, Balci MK, Altunbas H, et al. Clin Endocrinol (Oxf). 2003; 59: 258-62.

82. Sartorio A, Agosti F, Resnik M, et al. J Endocrinol Invest. 2003; 26: 250-6.

83. Scholz GH, Englaro P, Thiele I, et al. Horm Metab Res. 1996; 28: 718-23.

84. Soriano-Guillen L, Barrios V, Campos-Barros A, et al. J Pediatr. 2004; 144: 36-42.

85. Stokholm KH. Int J Obes. 1980; 4: 133-8.

86. Stokholm KH, Hansen MS. Int J Obes. 1983; 7: 195-9.

87. Sudi KM, Gallistl S, Borkenstein MH, et al. Endocrine. 2001; 14: 429-35.

88. Tereshchenko IV, Demicheva TP, Kashkina NV. Vopr Pitan. 1994; (3): 45-9.

89. Torgerson JS, Carlsson B, Stenlof K, et al. J Clin Endocrinol Metab. 1999; 84: 4197-203.

90. Turcato E, Zamboni M, De Pergola G, et al. J Intern Med. 1997; 241: 363-72.

91. van Gemert WG, Westerterp KR, van Acker BA, et al. Int J Obes Relat Metab Disord. 2000; 24: 711-8.

92. van Rossum EF, Nicklas BJ, Dennis KE, et al. Obes Res. 2000; 8: 29-35.

93. Verdich C, Toubro S, Buemann B, et al. Obes Res. 2001; 9: 452-61.

94. Verrotti A, Basciani F, De Simone M, et al. Diabetes Nutr Metab. 2001; 14: 283-7.

95. Visser TJ, Lamberts SW, Wilson JH, et al. Metabolism. 1978; 27: 405-9.

96. Wabitsch M, Hauner H, Heinze E, et al. J Clin Endocrinol Metab. 1995; 80: 3469-75.

97. Wadden TA, Considine RV, Foster GD, et al. J Clin Endocrinol Metab. 1998; 83: 214-8.

98. Wadden TA, Mason G, Foster GD, et al. Int J Obes. 1990; 14: 249-58.

99. Weigle DS, Duell PB, Connor WE, et al. J Clin Endocrinol Metab. 1997; 82: 561–565.

100. Wilkin TJ, Choquet RC, Schmouker Y, et al. Acta Endocrinol (Copenh). 1983; 103: 184-7.

101. Williams KV, Mullen M, Lang W, et al. Obes Res. 1999; 7: 155-63.

102. Wilson JH, Lamberts SW. Int J Obes. 1981; 5: 275-8.

103. Wing RR, Sinha MK, Considine RV, et al. Horm Metab Res. 1996; 28: 698-703.

104. Wisse BE, Campfield LA, Marliss EB, et al. Am J Clin Nutr. 1999; 70: 321-30.

105. Woodward CJ, Hervey GR, Oakey RE, et al. Br J Nutr. 1991; 66: 117-27.

106. Yip I, Go VL, Hershman JM, et al. Pancreas. 2001; 23: 197-203.

G

1. Anderson DA, Shapiro JR, Lundgren JD, et al. Appetite. 2002; 38: 13-7.

2. Anderson IM, Crook WS, Gartside SE, et al. J Affect Disord. 1989; 16(2-3): 197-202.

3. Goodwin GM, Fairburn CG, Keenan JC, et al. J Affect Disord. 1988; 14: 137-44.

4. Johnstone AM, Faber P, Andrew R, et al. Eur J Endocrinol. 2004; 150: 185-94.

5. McLean JA, Barr SI, Prior JC. Am J Clin Nutr. 2001; 73: 7-12.

H

1. Anderson IM, Crook WS, Gartside SE, et al. J Affect Disord. 1989; 16(2-3): 197-202.

2. Askari H, Liu J, Dagogo-Jack S. Int J Obes Relat Metab Disord. 2000; 24: 1254-9.

3. Beaufrere B, Horber FF, Schwenk WF, et al. Am J Physiol. 1989; 257(5 Pt 1): E712-21.

4. Bennet WM, Haymond MW. Clin Endocrinol (Oxf). 1992; 36: 161-4.

5. Berneis K, Ninnis R, Girard J, et al. J Clin Endocrinol Metab. 1997; 82: 2528-34.

6. Born J, Kern W, Bieber K, et al. Biol Psychiatry. 1986; 21: 1415-24.

7. Bornstein SR, Licinio J, Tauchnitz R, et al. J Clin Endocrinol Metab. 1998; 83: 280-3.

8. Chai J, Shen C, Sheng Z. Zhonghua Wai Ke Za Zhi. 2002; 40: 705-8.

9. Challet E, le Maho Y, Robin JP, et al. Pharmacol Biochem Behav. 1995; 50: 405-12.

10. Condren RM, O'Neill A, Ryan MC, et al. Psychoneuroendocrinology. 2002; 27: 693-703.

11. Crowley MA, Matt KS. Eur J Appl Physiol Occup Physiol. 1996; 73(1-2): 66-72.

12. Dagogo-Jack S, Umamaheswaran I, Askari H, et al. Obes Res. 2003; 11: 232-7.

13. Darmaun D, Matthews DE, Bier DM. Am J Physiol. 1988; 255(3 Pt 1): E366-73.

14. Deak T, Nguyen KT, Cotter CS, et al. Brain Res. 1999; 847: 211-20.

15. Deuster PA, Chrousos GP, Luger A, et al. Metabolism. 1989; 38: 141-8.

16. Deuster PA, Petrides JS, Singh A, et al. J Clin Endocrinol Metab. 1998; 83: 3332-8.

17. Devenport L, Knehans A, Sundstrom A, et al. Life Sci. 1989; 45: 1389-96.

18. Dickerson SS, Kemeny ME. Psychol Bull. 2004; 130: 355-91.

19. Dinneen S, Alzaid A, Miles J, et al. J Clin Invest. 1993; 92: 2283-90.

20. Dinneen S, Alzaid A, Miles J, et al. Am J Physiol. 1995; 268(4 Pt 1): E595-603.

21. Divertie GD, Jensen MD, Miles JM. Diabetes. 1991; 40: 1228-32.

22. Djurhuus CB, Gravholt CH, Nielsen S, et al. Am J Physiol Endocrinol Metab. 2002; 283: E172-7.

23. Djurhuus CB, Gravholt CH, Nielsen S, et al. Am J Physiol Endocrinol Metab. 2004; 286: E488-94.

24. Doman J, Thompson S, Grochocinski V, et al. Psychoneuroendocrinology. 1986; 11: 359-66.

25. Duclos M, Corcuff JB, Rashedi M, et al. Eur J Appl Physiol Occup Physiol. 1997; 75: 343-50.

26. Edwards S, Evans P, Hucklebridge F, et al. Psychoneuroendocrinology. 2001; 26: 613-22.

27. Epel E, Lapidus R, McEwen B, et al. Psychoneuroendocrinology. 2001; 26: 37-49.

28. Fain JN. Inhibition of glucose transport in fat cells and activation of lipolysis by glucocorticoids. In: Baxter JD, Rousseau GG, eds. Glucocorticoid hormone action. Berlin, Heidelberg, New York 1979:Springer-Verlag;547-560.

29. Fehm HL, Klein E, Holl R, et al. J Clin Endocrinol Metab. 1984; 58: 410-4.

30. Ferrando AA, Stuart CA, Sheffield-Moore M, et al. J Clin Endocrinol Metab. 1999; 84: 3515-21.

31. Fleshner M, Deak T, Spencer RL, et al. Endocrinology. 1995; 136: 5336-42.

32. Gaab J, Blattler N, Menzi T, et al. Psychoneuroendocrinology. 2003; 28: 767-79.

33. Gemmill ME, Eskay RL, Hall NL, et al. J Nutr. 2003; 133: 504-9.

34. Gerra G, Zaimovic A, Mascetti GG, et al. Psychoneuroendocrinology. 2001; 26: 91-107.

35. Gravholt CH, Dall R, Christiansen JS, et al. Obes Res. 2002; 10: 774-81.

36. Grossi G, Perski A, Lundberg U, et al. Integr Physiol Behav Sci. 2001; 36: 205-19.

37. Heikkonen E, Ylikahri R, Roine R, et al. Alcohol Clin Exp Res. 1996; 20: 711-6.

38. Hindmarsh KW, Tan L, Sankaran K, et al. West J Med. 1989; 151: 153-6.

39. Hoogeveen AR, Zonderland ML. Int J Sports Med. 1996; 17: 423-8.

40. Horber FF, Marsh HM, Haymond MW. Diabetes. 1991; 40: 141-9.

41. Kirschbaum C, Prussner JC, Stone AA, et al. Psychosom Med. 1995; 57: 468-74.

42. Kirschbaum C, Wust S, Hellhammer D. Psychosom Med. 1992; 54: 648-57.

43. Kuoppasalmi K, Naveri H, Harkonen M, et al. Scand J Clin Lab Invest. 1980; 40: 403-9.

44. Liu Z, Jahn LA, Long W, et al. J Clin Endocrinol Metab. 2001; 86: 2136-43.

45. Lofberg E, Gutierrez A, Wernerman J, et al. Eur J Clin Invest. 2002; 32: 345-53.

46. Louard RJ, Bhushan R, Gelfand RA, et al. J Clin Endocrinol Metab. 1994; 79: 278-84.

47. Luger A, Deuster PA, Kyle SB, et al. N Engl J Med. 1987; 316: 1309-15.

48. Martinek L, Oberascher-Holzinger K, Weishuhn S, et al. Neuro Endocrinol Lett. 2003; 24: 449-53.

49. Masuzaki H, Ogawa Y, Hosoda K, et al. J Clin Endocrinol Metab. 1997; 82: 2542-7.

50. May RC, Bailey JL, Mitch WE, et al. Kidney Int. 1996; 49: 679-83.

51. Moukas M, Vassiliou MP, Amygdalou A, et al. Clin Nutr. 2002; 21: 297-302.

52. Nagata S, Takeda F, Kurosawa M, et al. Equine Vet J Suppl. 1999; 30: 570-4.

53. Newcomer JW, Selke G, Melson AK, et al. Arch Gen Psychiatry. 1998; 55: 995-1000.

54. Nishiyama M, Makino S, Suemaru S, et al. Horm Res. 2000; 54: 69-73.

55. Papanicolaou DA, Mullen N, Kyrou I, et al. J Clin Endocrinol Metab. 2002; 87: 4515-21.

56. Petrides JS, Gold PW, Mueller GP, et al. J Appl Physiol. 1997; 82: 1979-88.

57. Petrides JS, Mueller GP, Kalogeras KT, et al. J Clin Endocrinol Metab. 1994; 79: 377-83.

58. Quan ZY, Walser M. Metabolism. 1991; 40: 1263-7.

59. Rebuffe-Scrive M, Lonnroth P, Andersson B, et al. J Obes Weight Regul. 1988; 7: 22-33.

60. Roglic G, Pibernik-Okanovic M, Prasek M, et al. Behav Med. 1993; 19: 53-9.

61. Samra JS, Clark ML, Humphreys SM, et al. Am J Physiol. 1996; 271(6 Pt 1): E996-1002.

62. Santidrian S, Marchon P, Zhao XH, et al. Growth. 1981; 45: 342-50.

63. Santidrian S, Young VR. Rev Esp Fisiol. 1980; 36: 205-14.

64. Savary I, Debras E, Dardevet D, et al. Br J Nutr. 1998; 79: 297-304.

65. Schmidt-Reinwald A, Pruessner JC, Hellhammer DH, et al. Life Sci. 1999; 64: 1653-60.

66. Scott RS, Scandrett MS. Diabetes Care. 1981; 4: 514-8.

67. Sheridan JF, Stark JL, Avitsur R, et al. Ann N Y Acad Sci. 2000; 917: 894-905.

68. Simmons PS, Miles JM, Gerich JE, et al. J Clin Invest. 1984; 73: 412-20.

69. Singh A, Petrides JS, Gold PW, et al. J Clin Endocrinol Metab. 1999; 84: 1944-8.

70. Smith AP. Nutr Neurosci. 2002; 5: 141-4.

71. Tan JT, Patel BK, Kaplan LM, et al. Endocrine. 1998; 8: 85-92.

72. Traustadottir T, Bosch PR, Matt KS. Stress. 2003; 6: 133-40.

73. Trumper BG, Reschke K, Molling J. Horm Metab Res. 1995; 27: 141-7.

74. Tyndall GL, Kobe RW, Houmard JA. Eur J Appl Physiol Occup Physiol. 1996; 73(1-2): 61-5.

75. Wittert GA, Livesey JH, Espiner EA, et al. Med Sci Sports Exerc. 1996; 28: 1015-9.

76. Wittert GA, Stewart DE, Graves MP, et al. Clin Endocrinol (Oxf). 1991; 35: 311-7.

I

1. Bujalska IJ, Kumar S, Hewison M, et al. Endocrinology. 1999; 140: 3188-96.

2. Gregoire F, Genart C, Hauser N, et al. Exp Cell Res. 1991; 196: 270-8.

3. Hauner H, Entenmann G, Wabitsch M, et al. J Clin Invest. 1989; 84: 1663-70.

4. Hauner H, Schmid P, Pfeiffer EF. J Clin Endocrinol Metab. 1987; 64: 832-5.

5. Hentges EJ, Hausman GJ. Domest Anim Endocrinol. 1989; 6: 275-85.

6. Nougues J, Reyne Y, Barenton B, et al. Int J Obes Relat Metab Disord. 1993; 17: 159-67.

7. Ramsay TG, White ME, Wolverton CK. J Anim Sci. 1989; 67: 2222-9.

8. Suryawan A, Swanson LV, Hu CY. J Anim Sci. 1997; 75: 105-11.

9. Xu XF, Bjorntorp P. Exp Cell Res. 1990; 189: 247-52.

J

1. Astrup A, Quaade F. Int J Obes. 1989; 13 Suppl 2: 27-31.

2. Doucet E, Tremblay A, Simoneau JA, et al. Am J Clin Nutr. 2003; 78: 430-5.

3. Dulloo AG, Girardier L. Metabolism. 1992; 41: 1336-42.

4. Dulloo AG, Jacquet J, Girardier L. Int J Obes Relat Metab Disord. 1996; 20: 393-405.

5. Ilagan J, Bhutani V, Archer P, et al. J Appl Physiol. 1993; 74: 2092-8.

6. Mingrone G, Marino S, DeGaetano A, et al. Metabolism. 2001; 50: 1004-7.

7. Votruba SB, Blanc S, Schoeller DA. Am J Physiol Endocrinol Metab. 2002; 282: E923-30.

K

1. Burstein R, Prentice AM, Goldberg GR, et al. Int J Obes Relat Metab Disord. 1996; 20: 253-9.

2. Fitzwater SL, Weinsier RL, Wooldridge NH, et al. J Am Diet Assoc. 1991; 91: 421-6, 429.

3. Fujimoto K, Sakata T, Etou H, et al. Am J Med Sci. 1992; 303: 145-50.

4. Hensrud DD, Weinsier RL, Darnell BE, et al. Obes Res. 1995; 3 Suppl 2: 217s-222s.

5. Hensrud DD, Weinsier RL, Darnell BE, et al. Am J Clin Nutr. 1994; 60: 688-94.

6. Kopec E, Widecka K, Krzyzanowska-Swiniarska B, et al. Pol Arch Med Wewn. 2004; 112: 1047-54.

7. Mavri A, Stegnar M, Sabovic M. Diabetes Obes Metab. 2001; 3: 293-6.

8. Mitsuhashi E, Lee JS, Kawakubo K. Nippon Koshu Eisei Zasshi. 2003; 50: 136-45.

9. Shepherd TM. J Fam Pract. 2003; 52: 34-42.

Problems With What We've Been Trying

A

1. Burgess NS. J Am Diet Assoc. 1991; 91: 430-4.

2. Capani F, De Luca C, Trapani F, et al. Boll Soc Ital Biol Sper. 1985; 61: 441-4.

3. Carella MJ, Rodgers CD, Anderson D, et al. Obes Res. 1997; 5: 250-6.

4. Coxon A, Kreitzman S, Brodie D, et al. Int J Obes. 1989; 13 Suppl 2: 179-81.

5. Dengel DR, Hagberg JM, Coon PJ, et al. Metabolism. 1994; 43: 867-71.

6. Deurenberg P, Weststrate JA, Hautvast JG. Am J Clin Nutr. 1989; 49: 33-6.

7. Deurenberg P, Weststrate JA, van der Kooy K. Am J Clin Nutr. 1989; 49: 401-3.

8. Donnelly JE, Jacobsen DJ, Whatley JE. Am J Clin Nutr. 1994; 60: 874-8.

9. Dulloo AG, Jacquet J, Girardier L. Int J Obes Relat Metab Disord. 1996; 20: 393-405.

10. Gallagher D, Kovera AJ, Clay-Williams G, et al. Am J Physiol Endocrinol Metab. 2000; 279: E124-31.

11. Hendel HW, Gotfredsen A, Hojgaard L, et al. Scand J Clin Lab Invest. 1996; 56: 671-9.

12. Johnson MJ, Friedl KE, Frykman PN, et al. Med Sci Sports Exerc. 1994; 26: 235-40.

13. Kruger J, Galuska DA, Serdula MK, et al. Am J Prev Med. 2004; 26: 402-6.

14. Morgan WD, Ryde SJ, Birks JL, et al. Am J Clin Nutr. 1992; 56(1 Suppl): 262S-264S.

15. Pachocka L. Rocz Panstw Zakl Hig. 1999; 50: 445-54.

16. Ross R, Leger L, Marliss EB, et al. Int J Obes. 1991; 15: 733-9.

17. Saunders NH, al-Zeibak S, Ryde SJ, et al. Int J Obes Relat Metab Disord. 1993; 17: 317-22.

18. Schwingshandl J, Sudi K, Eibl B, et al. Arch Dis Child. 1999; 81: 426-8.

19. Torigoe K, Numata O, Matsunaga M, et al. Acta Paediatr Jpn. 1997; 39: 28-33.

20. Valtuena S, Blanch S, Barenys M, et al. Int J Obes Relat Metab Disord. 1995; 19: 119-25.

21. van der Kooy K, Leenen R, Deurenberg P, et al. Int J Obes Relat Metab Disord. 1992; 16: 675-83.

22. Vaswani AN, Vartsky D, Ellis KJ, et al. Metabolism. 1983; 32: 185-8.

23. Wadden TA, Foster GD, Stunkard AJ, et al. Int J Eat Disord. 1996; 19: 5-12.

B

1. Adami S, Ferrari M, Galvanini G, et al. J Endocrinol Invest. 1979; 2: 271-4.

2. Barrows K, Snook JT. Am J Clin Nutr. 1987; 45: 391-8.

3. Bergendahl M, Vance ML, Iranmanesh A, et al. J Clin Endocrinol Metab. 1996; 81: 692-9.

4. Burgess NS. J Am Diet Assoc. 1991; 91: 430-4.

5. Cameron JL, Weltzin TE, McConaha C, et al. J Clin Endocrinol Metab. 1991; 73: 35-41.

6. Cavallo E, Armellini F, Zamboni M, et al. Horm Metab Res. 1990; 22: 632-5.

7. Chomard P, Vernhes G, Autissier N, et al. Eur J Clin Nutr. 1988; 42: 285-93.

8. Davies HJ, Baird IM, Fowler J, et al. Am J Clin Nutr. 1989; 49: 745-51.

9. Doucet E, St Pierre S, Almeras N, et al. J Clin Endocrinol Metab. 2000; 85: 1550-6.

10. Dulloo AG, Jacquet J. Am J Clin Nutr. 1998; 68: 599-606.

11. Froidevaux F, Schutz Y, Christin L, et al. Am J Clin Nutr. 1993; 57: 35-42.

12. Garrel DR, Todd KS, Pugeat MM, et al. Am J Clin Nutr. 1984; 39: 930-6.

13. Grant AM, Edwards OM, Howard AN, et al. Clin Endocrinol (Oxf). 1978; 9: 227-31.

14. Karklin A, Driver HS, Buffenstein R. Am J Clin Nutr. 1994; 59: 346-9.

15. Keim NL, Stern JS, Havel PJ. Am J Clin Nutr. 1998; 68: 794-801.

16. Kiortsis DN, Durack I, Turpin G. Eur J Pediatr. 1999; 158: 446-50.

17. Luke A, Schoeller DA. Metabolism. 1992; 41: 450-6.

18. Menozzi R, Bondi M, Baldini A, et al. Br J Nutr. 2000; 84: 515-20.

19. Miyawaki T, Masuzaki H, Ogawa Y, et al. Eur J Clin Nutr. 2002; 56: 593-600.

20. Nelson KM, Weinsier RL, James LD, et al. Am J Clin Nutr. 1992; 55: 924-33.

21. Pelletier C, Doucet E, Imbeault P, et al. Toxicol Sci. 2002; 67: 46-51.

22. Racette SB, Kohrt WM, Landt M, et al. Am J Clin Nutr. 1997; 66: 33-7.

23. Samuels MH, Kramer P. J Clin Endocrinol Metab. 1996; 81: 32-6.

24. Tereshchenko IV, Demicheva TP, Kashkina NV. Vopr Pitan. 1994; (3): 45-9.

25. van Gemert WG, Westerterp KR, van Acker BA, et al. Int J Obes Relat Metab Disord. 2000; 24: 711-8.

26. Wilkin TJ, Choquet RC, Schmouker Y, et al. Acta Endocrinol (Copenh). 1983; 103: 184-7.

27. Williams KV, Mullen M, Lang W, et al. Obes Res. 1999; 7: 155-63.

28. Wisse BE, Campfield LA, Marliss EB, et al. Am J Clin Nutr. 1999; 70: 321-30.

C

1. Klem ML, Wing RR, McGuire MT, et al. Am J Clin Nutr. 1997; 66: 239-46.
2. McGuire MT, Wing RR, Klem ML, et al. Obes Res. 1999; 7: 334-41.
3. McGuire MT, Wing RR, Klem ML, et al. Int J Obes Relat Metab Disord. 1998; 22: 572-7.
4. Shick SM, Wing RR, Klem ML, et al. J Am Diet Assoc. 1998; 98: 408-13.
5. Toubro S, Astrup AV. Ugeskr Laeger. 1998; 160: 816-20.

D

1. Astrup A. Curr Opin Clin Nutr Metab Care. 1998; 1: 573-7.
2. Astrup A, Toubro S, Raben A, et al. J Am Diet Assoc. 1997; 97(7 Suppl): S82-7.
3. Baron JA, Schori A, Crow B, et al. Am J Public Health. 1986; 76: 1293-6.
4. Brehm BJ, Seeley RJ, Daniels SR, et al. J Clin Endocrinol Metab. 2003; 88: 1617-23.
5. Djuric Z, Lababidi S, Heilbrun LK, et al. J Am Coll Nutr. 2002; 21: 38-46.
6. Flegal KM, Carroll MD, Kuczmarski RJ, et al. Int J Obes Relat Metab Disord. 1998; 22: 39-47.
7. Flegal KM, Carroll MD, Ogden CL, et al. JAMA. 2002; 288: 1723-7.
8. Galuska DA, Serdula M, Pamuk E, et al. Am J Public Health. 1996; 86: 1729-35.
9. Golay A, Eigenheer C, Morel Y, et al. Int J Obes Relat Metab Disord. 1996; 20: 1067-72.
10. Harvey-Berino J. Obes Res. 1998; 6: 202-7.
11. Heini AF, Weinsier RL. Am J Med. 1997; 102: 259-64.
12. Jeffery RW, Hellerstedt WL, French SA, et al. Int J Obes Relat Metab Disord. 1995; 19: 132-7.
13. Kuczmarski RJ, Flegal KM, Campbell SM, et al. The National Health and Nutrition Examination Surveys, 1960 to 1991. 1994; 272: 205-11.
14. McManus K, Antinoro L, Sacks F. Int J Obes Relat Metab Disord. 2001; 25: 1503-11.
15. Meckling KA, O'Sullivan C, Saari D. J Clin Endocrinol Metab. 2004; 89: 2717-23.
16. Ogden CL, Flegal KM, Carroll MD, et al. JAMA. 2002; 288: 1728-32.
17. Okosun IS, Chandra KM, Boev A, et al. Prev Med. 2004; 39: 197-206.
18. Pelkman CL, Fishell VK, Maddox DH, et al. Am J Clin Nutr. 2004; 79: 204-12.
19. Rock CL, Thomson C, Caan BJ, et al. Cancer. 2001; 91: 25-34.
20. Rodriguez Artalejo F, Lopez Garcia E, Gutierrez-Fisac JL, et al. Prev Med. 2002; 34: 72-81.
21. Schlundt DG, Hill JO, Pope-Cordle J, et al. Int J Obes Relat Metab Disord. 1993; 17: 623-9.
22. Seim HC, Holtmeier KB. Fam Pract Res J. 1992; 12: 411-9.
23. Sheppard L, Kristal AR, Kushi LH. Am J Clin Nutr. 1991; 54: 821-8.
24. Silventoinen K, Sans S, Tolonen H, et al. Int J Obes Relat Metab Disord. 2004; 28: 710-8.
25. Thomson CA, Rock CL, Giuliano AR, et al. Eur J Nutr. 2005; 44: 18-25.
26. Urban N, White E, Anderson GL, et al. Prev Med. 1992; 21: 279-91.
27. Willett WC, Leibel RL. Am J Med. 2002; 113 Suppl 9B: 47S-59S.

E

1. Baron JA, Schori A, Crow B, et al. Am J Public Health. 1986; 76: 1293-6.
2. McManus K, Antinoro L, Sacks F. Int J Obes Relat Metab Disord. 2001; 25: 1503-11.
3. Pritchard JE, Nowson CA, Wark JD. J Am Diet Assoc. 1997; 97: 37-42.
4. Schlundt DG, Hill JO, Pope-Cordle J, et al. Int J Obes Relat Metab Disord. 1993; 17: 623-9.

F

1. Abbasi F, McLaughlin T, Lamendola C, et al. Am J Cardiol. 2000; 85: 45-8.

2. Abbott WG, Boyce VL, Grundy SM, et al. Diabetes Care. 1989; 12: 102-7.

3. Anderson JW. Can Med Assoc J. 1980; 123: 975-9.

4. Anderson JW, Garrity TF, Wood CL, et al. Am J Clin Nutr. 1992; 56: 887-94.

5. Baron JA, Schori A, Crow B, et al. Am J Public Health. 1986; 76: 1293-6.

6. Borkman M, Campbell LV, Chisholm DJ, et al. J Clin Endocrinol Metab. 1991; 72: 432-7.

7. Brehm BJ, Seeley RJ, Daniels SR, et al. J Clin Endocrinol Metab. 2003; 88: 1617-23.

8. Carmichael HE, Swinburn BA, Wilson MR. J Am Diet Assoc. 1998; 98: 35-9.

9. Chen YD, Coulston AM, Zhou MY, et al. Diabetes Care. 1995; 18: 10-6.

10. Clevidence BA, Judd JT, Schatzkin A, et al. Am J Clin Nutr. 1992; 55: 689-94.

11. Coulston AM, Hollenbeck CB, Swislocki AL, et al. Am J Med. 1987; 82: 213-20.

12. Coulston AM, Hollenbeck CB, Swislocki AL, et al. Diabetes Care. 1989; 12: 94-101.

13. Coulston AM, Liu GC, Reaven GM. Metabolism. 1983; 32: 52-6.

14. Denke MA, Breslow JL. J Lipid Res. 1988; 29: 963-9.

15. Djuric Z, Lababidi S, Heilbrun LK, et al. J Am Coll Nutr. 2002; 21: 38-46.

16. Dreon DM, Fernstrom HA, Williams PT, et al. Am J Clin Nutr. 1999; 69: 411-8.

17. Fuh MM, Lee MM, Jeng CY, et al. Am J Hypertens. 1990; 3: 527-32.

18. Fukita Y, Gott o AM, Unger RH. Diabetes. 1975; 24: 552-8.

19. Garg A, Grundy SM, Koffler M. Diabetes Care. 1992; 15: 1572-80.

20. Ginsberg H, Olefsky JM, Kimmerling G, et al. J Clin Endocrinol Metab. 1976; 42: 729-35.

21. Golay A, Eigenheer C, Morel Y, et al. Int J Obes Relat Metab Disord. 1996; 20: 1067-72.

22. Grundy SM. N Engl J Med. 1986; 314: 745-8.

23. Hagenfeldt L, Hellstrom K, Wahren J. Clin Sci Mol Med. 1975; 48: 247-57.

24. Harris WS, Connor WE, Inkeles SB, et al. Metabolism. 1984; 33: 1016-9.

25. Harvey-Berino J. Obes Res. 1998; 6: 202-7.

26. Hudgins LC, Hellerstein MK, Seidman CE, et al. J Lipid Res. 2000; 41: 595-604.

27. Jacobs B, De Angelis-Schierbaum G, Egert S, et al. J Nutr. 2004; 134: 1400-5.

28. Jeffery RW, Hellerstedt WL, French SA, et al. Int J Obes Relat Metab Disord. 1995; 19: 132-7.

29. Jeppesen J, Schaaf P, Jones C, et al. Am J Clin Nutr. 1997; 66: 437.

30. Judd JT, Oh SY, Hennig B, et al. J Am Coll Nutr. 1988; 7: 223-34.

31. Julius U, Schulze J, Schollberg K, et al. Endokrinologie. 1978; 71: 299-307.

32. Kasim-Karakas SE, Almario RU, Mueller WM, et al. Am J Clin Nutr. 2000; 71: 1439-47.

33. Koutsari C, Malkova D, Hardman AE. Metabolism. 2000; 49: 1150-5.

34. Krauss RM, Dreon DM. Am J Clin Nutr. 1995; 62: 478S-487S.

35. Leddy J, Horvath P, Rowland J, et al. Med Sci Sports Exerc. 1997; 29: 17-25.

36. Liu B, He Y, Zhang R, et al. Hua Xi Yi Ke Da Xue Xue Bao. 1990; 21: 145-9.

37. Liu G, Coulston A, Hollenbeck C, et al. J Clin Endocrinol Metab. 1984; 59: 636-42.

38. Liu GC, Coulston AM, Reaven GM. Metabolism. 1983; 32: 750-3.

39. Louheranta AM, Schwab US, Sarkkinen ES, et al. Nutr Metab Cardiovasc Dis. 2000; 10: 177-87.

40. Marckmann P, Sandstrom B, Jespersen J. Am J Clin Nutr. 1994; 59: 935-9.

41. Marques-Lopes I, Ansorena D, Astiasaran I, et al. Am J Clin Nutr. 2001; 73: 253-61.

42. McLaughlin T, Abbasi F, Lamendola C, et al. J Clin Endocrinol Metab. 2000; 85: 3085-8.

43. McManus K, Antinoro L, Sacks F. Int J Obes Relat Metab Disord. 2001; 25: 1503-11.

44. Meckling KA, O'Sullivan C, Saari D. J Clin Endocrinol Metab. 2004; 89: 2717-23.

45. Mirani-Oostdijk CP, van Gent CM, Terpstra J, et al. Acta Med Scand. 1981; 210: 277-82.

46. Mohanlal N, Holman RR. Diabetes Care. 2004; 27: 89-94.

47. Mueller-Cunningham WM, Quintana R, Kasim-Karakas SE. J Am Diet Assoc. 2003; 103: 1600-6.

48. Nolan CJ. Aust N Z J Obstet Gynaecol. 1984; 24: 174-7.

49. O'Brien T, Nguyen TT, Buithieu J, et al. J Clin Endocrinol Metab. 1993; 77: 1345-51.

50. O'Dea K, Traianedes K, Ireland P, et al. J Am Diet Assoc. 1989; 89: 1076-86.

51. Olefsky JM, Crapo P, Reaven GM. Am J Clin Nutr. 1976; 29: 535-9.

52. Parillo M, Coulston A, Hollenbeck C, et al. Hypertension. 1988; 11: 244-8.

53. Parks EJ, Rutledge JC, Davis PA, et al. J Cardiopulm Rehabil. 2001; 21: 73-9.

54. Pelkman CL, Fishell VK, Maddox DH, et al. Am J Clin Nutr. 2004; 79: 204-12.

55. Poppitt SD, Keogh GF, Prentice AM, et al. Am J Clin Nutr. 2002; 75: 11-20.

56. Raben A, Jensen ND, Marckmann P, et al. Int J Obes Relat Metab Disord. 1995; 19: 916-23.

57. Sacks FM, Handysides GH, Marais GE, et al. Arch Intern Med. 1986; 146: 1573-7.

58. Sanchez E, Jansen S, Castro P, et al. Med Clin (Barc). 1999; 112: 206-10.

59. Sanfelippo ML, Swenson RS, Reaven GM. Kidney Int. 1977; 11: 54-61.

60. Santos MS, Lichtenstein AH, Leka LS, et al. J Am Coll Nutr. 2003; 22: 174-82.

61. Schaefer EJ, Lamon-Fava S, Spiegelman D, et al. Metabolism. 1995; 44: 749-56.

62. Schaefer EJ, Levy RI, Ernst ND, et al. Am J Clin Nutr. 1981; 34: 1758-63.

63. Schlundt DG, Hill JO, Pope-Cordle J, et al. Int J Obes Relat Metab Disord. 1993; 17: 623-9.

64. Seim HC, Holtmeier KB. Fam Pract Res J. 1992; 12: 411-9.

65. Shah M, McGovern P, French S, et al. Am J Clin Nutr. 1994; 59: 980-4.

66. Sheppard L, Kristal AR, Kushi LH. Am J Clin Nutr. 1991; 54: 821-8.

67. Siggaard R, Raben A, Astrup A. Obes Res. 1996; 4: 347-56.

68. Silaste ML, Rantala M, Alfthan G, et al. Arterioscler Thromb Vasc Biol. 2004; 24: 498-503.

69. Snook JT, DeLany JP, Vivian VM. Lipids. 1985; 20: 808-16.

70. Stasse-Wolthuis M, Hautvast JG, Hermus RJ, et al. Am J Clin Nutr. 1979; 32: 1881-8.

71. Straznicky NE, O'Callaghan CJ, Barrington VE, et al. Hypertension. 1999; 34(4 Pt 1): 580-5.

72. Toubro S, Astrup A. BMJ. 1997; 314: 29-34.

73. Toubro S, Astrup AV. Ugeskr Laeger. 1998; 160: 816-20.

74. Turley ML, Skeaff CM, Mann JI, et al. Eur J Clin Nutr. 1998; 52: 728-32.

75. Ullmann D, Connor WE, Hatcher LF, et al. Arterioscler Thromb. 1991; 11: 1059-67.

G

1. Freeman JM, Vining EP, Pillas DJ, et al. Pediatrics. 1998; 102: 1358-63.

2. Katyal NG, Koehler AN, McGhee B, et al. Clin Pediatr (Phila). 2000; 39: 153-9.

3. Livingston S. Postgrad Med. 1951; 10: 333-6.

4. Musa-Veloso K, Rarama E, Comeau F, et al. Pediatr Res. 2002; 52: 443-8.

5. Thiele EA. Epilepsia. 2003; 44 Suppl 7: 26-9.

H

1. Astrup A, Buemann B, Christensen NJ, et al. Am J Physiol. 1994; 266(4 Pt 1): E592-9.

2. Baron JA, Schori A, Crow B, et al. Am J Public Health. 1986; 76: 1293-6.

3. Brehm BJ, Seeley RJ, Daniels SR, et al. J Clin Endocrinol Metab. 2003; 88: 1617-23.

4. Buemann B, Toubro S, Astrup A. Int J Obes Relat Metab Disord. 1998; 22: 869-77.

5. Elliot B, Roeser HP, Warrell A, et al. Med J Aust. 1981; 1: 237-40.

6. Foster GD, Wyatt HR, Hill JO, et al. N Engl J Med. 2003; 348: 2082-90.

7. Fukita Y, Gott o AM, Unger RH. Diabetes. 1975; 24: 552-8.

8. Golay A, Eigenheer C, Morel Y, et al. Int J Obes Relat Metab Disord. 1996; 20: 1067-72.

9. Lewis SB, Wallin JD, Kane JP, et al. Am J Clin Nutr. 1977; 30: 160-70.

10. Malewiak MI, Griglio S, Moulin N, et al. Biomedicine. 1977; 26: 297-302.

11. Meckling KA, Gauthier M, Grubb R, et al. Can J Physiol Pharmacol. 2002; 80: 1095-105.

12. Meckling KA, O'Sullivan C, Saari D. J Clin Endocrinol Metab. 2004; 89: 2717-23.

13. Rabast U, Kasper H, Schonborn J. Nutr Metab. 1978; 22: 269-77.

14. Rabast U, Schonborn J, Kasper H. Int J Obes. 1979; 3: 201-11.

15. Rabast U, Vornberger KH, Ehl M. Ann Nutr Metab. 1981; 25. 341-9.

16. Roy HJ, Lovejoy JC, Keenan MJ, et al. Am J Clin Nutr. 1998; 67: 405-11.

17. Samaha FF, Iqbal N, Seshadri P, et al. N Engl J Med. 2003; 348: 2074-81.

18. Schutz Y, Flatt JP, Jequier E. Am J Clin Nutr. 1989; 50: 307-14.

19. Sharman MJ, Gomez AL, Kraemer WJ, et al. J Nutr. 2004; 134: 880-5.

20. Sharman MJ, Volek JS. Clin Sci (Lond). 2004; 107: 365-9.

21. Smith SR, de Jonge L, Zachwieja JJ, et al. Am J Clin Nutr. 2000; 71: 450-7.

22. Sondike SB, Copperman N, Jacobson MS. J Pediatr. 2003; 142: 253-8.

23. Stern L, Iqbal N, Seshadri P, et al. Ann Intern Med. 2004; 140: 778-85.

24. Volek JS, Sharman MJ, Gomez AL, et al. J Am Coll Nutr. 2004; 23: 177-84.

25. Volek JS, Sharman MJ, Love DM, et al. Metabolism. 2002; 51: 864-70.

26. Westman EC, Yancy WS, Edman JS, et al. Am J Med. 2002; 113: 30-6.

27. Yancy WS Jr, Olsen MK, Guyton JR, et al. Ann Intern Med. 2004; 140: 769-77.

28. Yerboeket-van de Venne WP, Westerterp KR. Appetite. 1996; 26: 287-300.

I

1. Blake WL, Clarke SD. J Nutr. 1990; 120: 1727-9.

2. Boll M, Weber LW, Stampfl A. Z Naturforsch C. 1996; 51(11-12): 859-69.

3. Carrozza G, Livrea G, Caponetti R, et al. J Nutr. 1979; 109: 162-70.

4. Clarke SD, Armstrong MK, Jump DB. J Nutr. 1990; 120: 218-24.

5. Clarke SD, Armstrong MK, Jump DB. J Nutr. 1990; 120: 225-31.

6. Foufelle F, Perdereau D, Gouhot B, et al. Eur J Biochem. 1992; 208: 381-7.

7. Hill JO, Lin D, Yakubu F, et al. Int J Obes Relat Metab Disord. 1992; 16: 321-33.

8. Kim H, Choi S, Lee HJ, et al. J Biochem Mol Biol. 2003; 36: 258-64.

9. Morris KL, Namey TC, Zemel MB. J Nutr Biochem. 2003; 14: 32-9.

10. Shillabeer G, Hornford J, Forden JM, et al. J Lipid Res. 1990; 31: 623-31.

11. Shillabeer G, Hornford J, Forden JM, et al. J Lipid Res. 1992; 33: 31-9.

12. Wolf G. Nutr Rev. 1996; 54(4 Pt 1): 122-3.

J

1. Foster GD, Wyatt HR, Hill JO, et al. N Engl J Med. 2003; 348: 2082-90.

K

1. Arner P, Bolinder J, Ostman J. Science. 1983; 220: 1057-9.

2. Avogaro A, Valerio A, Gnudi L, et al. Diabetologia. 1992; 35: 129-38.

3. Boden G, Chen X, Desantis RA, et al. Diabetes. 1993; 42: 1588-93.

4. Bonadonna RC, Groop LC, Zych K, et al. Am J Physiol. 1990; 259(5 Pt 1): E736-50.

5. Burge MR, Hardy KJ, Schade DS. J Clin Endocrinol Metab. 1993; 76: 1192-8.

6. Campbell PJ, Carlson MG, Hill JO, et al. Am J Physiol. 1992; 263(6 Pt 1): E1063-9.

7. Capaldo B, Napoli R, Di Marino L, et al. J Clin Endocrinol Metab. 1994; 79: 879-82.

8. Cavallo-Perin P, Bruno A, Cassader M, et al. Eur J Clin Invest. 1992; 22: 725-31.

9. Coppack SW, Frayn KN, Humphreys SM, et al. Clin Sci (Lond). 1989; 77: 663-70.

10. Dyck DJ, Steinberg G, Bonen A. Am J Physiol Endocrinol Metab. 2001; 281: E600-7.

11. Enoksson S, Degerman E, Hagstrom-Toft E, et al. Diabetologia. 1998; 41: 560-8.

12. Goldrick RB, McLoughlin GM. J Clin Invest. 1970; 49: 1213-23.

13. Groop LC, Bonadonna RC, Simonson DC, et al. Am J Physiol. 1992; 263(1 Pt 1): E79-84.

14. Hammond VA, Johnston DG. Metabolism. 1987; 36: 308-13.

15. Howard BV, Klimes I, Vasquez B, et al. J Clin Endocrinol Metab. 1984; 58: 544-8.

16. Jacob S, Hauer B, Becker R, et al. Diabetologia. 1999; 42: 1171-4.

17. Jensen MD, Caruso M, Heiling V, et al. Diabetes. 1989; 38: 1595-601.

18. Jensen MD, Haymond MW, Gerich JE, et al. J Clin Invest. 1987; 79: 207-13.

19. Meek SE, Nair KS, Jensen MD. Diabetes. 1999; 48: 10-4.

20. Miles JM, Haymond MW, Gerich JE. Ciba Found Symp. 1982; 87: 192-213.

21. Muller-Hess R, Geser CA, Pittet P, et al. Diabete Metab. 1975; 1: 151-7.

22. Newsholme EA, Dimitriadis G. Exp Clin Endocrinol Diabetes. 2001; 109 Suppl 2: S122-34.

23. Nurjhan N, Campbell PJ, Kennedy FP, et al. Diabetes. 1986; 35: 1326-31.

24. Pimenta WP, Saad MJ, Paccola GM, et al. Braz J Med Biol Res. 1989; 22: 465-76.

25. Robinson C, Tamborlane WV, Maggs DG, et al. Am J Physiol. 1998; 274(4 Pt 1): E737-43.

26. Sidossis LS, Wolfe RR. Am J Physiol. 1996; 270(4 Pt 1): E733-8.

27. Stumvoll M, Jacob S, Wahl HG, et al. J Clin Endocrinol Metab. 2000; 85: 3740-5.

28. Townsend RR, Zhao H. Metabolism. 2002; 51: 779-82.

L

1. Anderwald C, Brabant G, Bernroider E, et al. Diabetes. 2003; 52: 1792-8.

2. Ashley DV, Liardon R, Leathwood PD. J Neural Transm. 1985; 63(3-4): 271-83.

3. Azar ST, Zalloua PA, Zantout MS, et al. J Endocrinol Invest. 2002; 25: 724-6.

4. Barr VA, Malide D, Zarnowski MJ, et al. Endocrinology. 1997; 138: 4463-72.

5. Bertin E, Rich N, Schneider N, et al. Diabetes Metab. 1998; 24: 229-34.

6. Bomboy JD, Lewis SB, Sinclair-Smith BC, et al. J Clin Endocrinol Metab. 1977; 44: 474-80.

7. Broglio F, Gottero C, Benso A, et al. J Clin Endocrinol Metab. 2003; 88: 4268-72.

8. Cammisotto PG, Bukowiecki LJ. Am J Physiol Cell Physiol. 2002; 283: C244-50.

9. Carey PE, Stewart MW, Ashworth L, et al. Horm Metab Res. 2003; 35: 372-6.

10. Casabiell X, Pineiro V, De la Cruz LF, et al. Biochem Biophys Res Commun. 2000; 276: 477-82.

11. Cherrington AD, Chiasson JL, Liljenquist JE, et al. J Clin Invest. 1976; 58: 1407-18.

12. Chiasson JL, Atkinson RL, Cherrington AD, et al. Metabolism. 1980; 29: 810-8.

13. Chiasson JL, Liljenquist JE, Finger FE, et al. Diabetes. 1976; 25: 283-91.

14. Couillard C, Mauriege P, Prud'homme D, et al. Diabetologia. 1997; 40: 1178-84.

15. Cuatrecasas G, Granada ML, Formiguera X, et al. Clin Endocrinol (Oxf). 1998; 48: 181-5.

16. Davis SN, Goldstein RE, Jacobs J, et al. Diabetes. 1993; 42: 263-72.

17. Fain JN, Cowan GS Jr, Buffington C, et al. Metabolism. 2000; 49: 804-9.

18. Fernstrom JD, Wurtman RJ. Science. 1971; 174: 1023-5.

19. Ferrannini E, DeFronzo RA, Sherwin RS. Am J Physiol. 1982; 242: E73-81.

20. Figlewicz DP, Sipols AJ, Seeley RJ, et al. Behav Neurosci. 1995; 109: 567-9.

21. Flanagan DE, Evans ML, Monsod TP, et al. Am J Physiol Endocrinol Metab. 2003; 284: E313-6.

22. Fluck CE, Kuhlmann BV, Mullis PE. Diabetologia. 1999; 42: 1067-70.

23. Giacca A, Fisher SJ, McCall RH, et al. Endocrinology. 1997; 138: 999-1007.

24. Giacca A, Fisher SJ, Shi ZQ, et al. J Clin Invest. 1992; 90: 1769-77.

25. Hanaki K, Becker DJ, Arslanian SA. J Clin Endocrinol Metab. 1999; 84: 1524-6.

26. Haqq AM, Farooqi IS, O'Rahilly S, et al. J Clin Endocrinol Metab. 2003; 88: 174-8.

27. Hasegawa H, Shirohara H, Okabayashi Y, et al. Metabolism. 1996; 45: 196-202.

28. Havel PJ, Uriu-Hare JY, Liu T, et al. Am J Physiol. 1998; 274(5 Pt 2): R1482-91.

29. Ito K, Maruyama H, Hirose H, et al. Metabolism. 1995; 44: 358-62.

30. Kirel B, Dogruel N, Korkmaz U, et al. Clin Biochem. 2000; 33: 475-80.

31. Kolaczynski JW, Nyce MR, Considine RV, et al. Diabetes. 1996; 45: 699-701.

32. Laferrere B, Caixas A, Fried SK, et al. Eur J Endocrinol. 2002; 146: 839-45.

33. Lavoie C, Ducros F, Bourque J, et al. Can J Physiol Pharmacol. 1997; 75: 26-35.

34. Lucidi P, Murdolo G, Di Loreto C, et al. Diabetes. 2002; 51: 2911-4.

35. Lyons PM, Truswell AS. Am J Clin Nutr. 1988; 47: 433-9.

36. McCowen KC, Maykel JA, Bistrian BR, et al. J Endocrinol. 2002; 175: R7-11.

37. Mohlig M, Spranger J, Otto B, et al. J Endocrinol Invest. 2002; 25: RC36-8.

38. Moller SE. Physiol Behav. 1986; 38: 175-83.

39. Murdolo G, Lucidi P, Di Loreto C, et al. Diabetes. 2003; 52: 2923-7.

40. Nagasaka S, Ishikawa S, Nakamura T, et al. Metabolism. 1998; 47: 1391-6.

41. Purnell JQ, Weigle DS, Breen P, et al. J Clin Endocrinol Metab. 2003; 88: 5747-52.

42. Riedy CA, Chavez M, Figlewicz DP, et al. Physiol Behav. 1995; 58: 755-60.

43. Russell CD, Petersen RN, Rao SP, et al. Am J Physiol. 1998; 275(3 Pt 1): E507-15.

44. Saad MF, Bernaba B, Hwu CM, et al. J Clin Endocrinol Metab. 2002; 87: 3997-4000.

45. Sacca L, Vitale D, Cicala M, et al. Metabolism. 1981; 30: 457-61.

46. Schaller G, Schmidt A, Pleiner J, et al. Diabetes. 2003; 52: 16-20.

47. Schmitz O, Fisker S, Orskov L, et al. Diabetes Metab. 1997; 23: 80-3.

48. Soriano-Guillen L, Barrios V, Lechuga-Sancho A, et al. Pediatr Res. 2004; 55: 830-5.

49. Stenvinkel P, Heimburger O, Lonnqvist F. Nephrol Dial Transplant. 1997; 12: 1321-5.

50. Stevenson RW, Williams PE, Cherrington AD. Diabetologia. 1987; 30: 782-90.

51. Tan JI, Patel BK, Kaplan LM, et al. Endocrine. 1998; 8: 85-92.

52. Utriainen T, Malmstrom R, Makimattila S, et al. Diabetes. 1996; 45: 1364-6.

53. Wabitsch M, Jensen PB, Blum WF, et al. Diabetes. 1996; 45: 1435-8.

54. Wurtman RJ, Wurtman JJ, Regan MM, et al. Am J Clin Nutr. 2003; 77: 128-32.

55. Yip I, Go VL, Hershman JM, et al. Pancreas. 2001; 23: 197-203.

M

1. Air EL, Strowski MZ, Benoit SC, et al. Nat Med. 2002; 8: 303.

2. Barba G, Russo O, Siani A, et al. Obes Res. 2003; 11: 160-6.

3. Benoit SC, Air EL, Coolen LM, et al. J Neurosci. 2002; 22: 9048-52.

4. Boyko EJ, Leonetti DL, Bergstrom RW, et al. Diabetes. 1996; 45: 1010-5.

5. Bruning JC, Gautam D, Burks DJ, et al. Science. 2000; 289: 2122-5.

6. Campfield LA, Smith FJ, Guisez Y, et al. Science. 1995; 269: 546-9.

7. Ceddia RB, William WN Jr, Lima FB, et al. J Endocrinol. 1998; 158: R7-9.

8. Ceddia RB, William WN Jr, Lima FB, et al. Eur J Biochem. 2000; 267: 5952-8.

9. Chapman IM, Goble EA, Wittert GA, et al. Am J Physiol. 1998; 274(3 Pt 2): R596-603.

10. Elias CF, Lee C, Kelly J, et al. Neuron. 1998; 21: 1375-85.

11. Elimam A, Kamel A, Marcus C. Horm Res. 2002; 58: 88-93.

12. Folsom AR, Vitelli LL, Lewis CE, et al. Int J Obes Relat Metab Disord. 1998; 22: 48-54.

13. Fraser DA, Thoen J, Bondhus S, et al. Clin Exp Rheumatol. 2000; 18: 209-14.

14. Fruhbeck G, Aguado M, Gomez-Ambrosi J, et al. Biochem Biophys Res Commun. 1998; 250: 99-102.

15. Fruhbeck G, Aguado M, Martinez JA. Biochem Biophys Res Commun. 1997; 240: 590-4.

16. Fruhbeck G, Gomez-Ambrosi J. Med Sci Monit. 2002; 8: BR47-55.

17. Fruhbeck G, Gomez-Ambrosi J, Salvador J. FASEB J. 2001; 15: 333-40.

18. Garcia-Lorda P, Bullo M, Vila R, et al. Diabetes Nutr Metab. 2001; 14: 329-36.

19. Gerozissis K. Eur J Pharmacol. 2004; 490(1-3): 59-70.

20. Gerozissis K, Kyriaki G. Cell Mol Neurobiol. 2003; 23(4-5): 873-4.

21. Halaas JL, Gajiwala KS, Maffei M, et al. Science. 1995; 269: 543-6.

22. Hickey MS, Considine RV, Israel RG, et al. Am J Physiol. 1996; 271(5 Pt 1): E938-40.

23. Hoag S, Marshall JA, Jones RH, et al. Int J Obes Relat Metab Disord. 1995; 19: 175-80.

24. Kamohara S, Burcelin R, Halaas JL, et al. Nature. 1997; 389: 374-7.

25. McMinn JE, Baskin DG, Schwartz MW. Obes Rev. 2000; 1: 37-46.

26. Mistry AM, Swick AG, Romsos DR. J Nutr. 1997; 127: 2065-72.

27. Morley JE, Alshaher MM, Farr SA, et al. Peptides. 1999; 20: 595-600.

28. Niswender KD, Schwartz MW. Front Neuroendocrinol. 2003; 24: 1-10.

29. Obici S, Feng Z, Karkanias G, et al. Nat Neurosci. 2002; 5: 566-72.

30. Pelleymounter MA, Cullen MJ, Baker MB, et al. Science. 1995; 269: 540-3.

31. Porte D Jr, Baskin DG, Schwartz MW. Nutr Rev. 2002; 60(10 Pt 2): S20-9; discussion S68-84, 85-7.

32. Porte D Jr, Woods SC. Diabetologia. 1981; 20 Suppl: 274-80.

33. Ramsay TG. J Anim Sci. 2003; 81: 3008-17.

34. Ramsay TG. J Anim Sci. 2001; 79: 653-7.

35. Ranganathan S, Maffei M, Kern PA. J Lipid Res. 1998; 39: 724-30.

36. Schwartz MW. Exp Biol Med (Maywood). 2001; 226: 978-81.

37. Schwartz MW, Boyko EJ, Kahn SE, et al. J Clin Endocrinol Metab. 1995; 80: 1571-6.

38. Siegrist-Kaiser CA, Pauli V, Juge-Aubry CE, et al. J Clin Invest. 1997; 100: 2858-64.

39. Wang MY, Lee Y, Unger RH. J Biol Chem. 1999; 274: 17541-4.

40. Wang ZW, Zhou YT, Lee Y, et al. Biochem Biophys Res Commun. 1999; 260: 653-7.

41. Weyer C, Hanson K, Bogardus C, et al. Diabetologia. 2000; 43: 36-46.

42. William WN Jr, Ceddia RB, Curi R. J Endocrinol. 2002; 175: 735-44.

43. Withers DJ. Biochem Soc Trans. 2001; 29(Pt 4): 525-9.

44. Woods SC, Chavez M, Park CR, et al. Neurosci Biobehav Rev. 1996; 20: 139-44.

45. Woods SC, Seeley RJ. Int J Obes Relat Metab Disord. 2001; 25 Suppl 5: S35-8.

46. Wozniak M, Rydzewski B, Baker SP, et al. Neurochem Int. 1993; 22: 1-10.

47. Zhang HH, Kumar S, Barnett AH, et al. J Clin Endocrinol Metab. 1999; 84: 2550-6.

N

1. Calle-Pascual AL, Gomez V, Leon E, et al. Diabete Metab. 1988; 14: 629-33.

2. Coulston AM, Reaven GM. Diabetes Care. 1997; 20: 241-3.

3. Monro J. J Nutr. 2003; 133: 4256-8.

4. Reaven GM. Curr Atheroscler Rep. 2000; 2: 503-7.

O

1. Berg G, Matzkies F, Heid H, et al. Z Ernahrungswiss. 1975; 14: 163-74.

2. Dallongeville J, Harbis A, Lebel P, et al. J Nutr. 2002; 132: 2161-6.

3. de Kalbermatten N, Ravussin E, Maeder E, et al. Metabolism. 1980; 29: 62-7.

4. Halperin ML, Cheema-Dhadli S. Biochem J. 1982; 202: 717-21.

5. Kazumi T, Vranic M, Steiner G. Am J Physiol. 1986; 250(3 Pt 1): E325-30.

6. Kazumi T, Yoshino G, Matsuba K, et al. Metabolism. 1991; 40: 962-6.

7. Pellaton M, Acheson K, Maeder E, et al. JPEN J Parenter Enteral Nutr. 1978; 2: 627-33.

8. Rawat AK, Menahan LA. Diabetes. 1975; 24: 926-32.

9. Rizkalla SW, Boillot J, Tricottet V, et al. Br J Nutr. 1993; 70: 199-209.

10. Rizkalla SW, Luo J, Guilhem I, et al. Mol Cell Biochem. 1992; 109: 127-32.

11. Schwarz JM, Neese RA, Basinger A, et al. FASEB J. 1993; 7: A867.

P

1. De Lorenzo A, Petroni ML, De Luca PP, et al. Diabetes Nutr Metab. 2001; 14: 181-8.

2. Elliott SS, Keim NL, Stern JS, et al. Am J Clin Nutr. 2002; 76: 911-22.

3. Fernandez de la Puebla RA, Fuentes F, Perez-Martinez P, et al. Nutr Metab Cardiovasc Dis. 2003; 13: 273-7.

4. Flynn G, Colquhoun D. Asia Pac J Clin Nutr. 2004; 13(Suppl): S139.

5. Fossati P. Ann Endocrinol (Paris). 1993; 54: 389-97.

6. Goodson S, Halford JC, Jackson HC, et al. Appetite. 2001; 37: 253-4.

7. Goulet J, Lamarche B, Nadeau G, et al. Atherosclerosis. 2003; 170: 115-24.

8. Havel PJ. Exp Clin Endocrinol Diabetes. 1997; 105: 37-38.

9. Havel PJ, Elliot SS, Tschoep M, et al. J Invest Med. 2002; 50: 26A (abstract).

10. Parks EJ. Br J Nutr. 2002; 87 Suppl 2: S247-53.

11. Parks EJ (2002) The relationship of the glycemic index to lipogenesis in humans. In Proceedings of the 6th (Millennium). Vahouny Conference D Kritchevsky, editor.. New York: Kluwer/Plenum Press.

12. Saris WH. Am J Clinical Nutrition. 2003; 78: 850S - 857.

13. Schwartz MW, Boyko EJ, Kahn SE, et al. J Clin Endocrinol Metab. 1995; 80: 1571-6.

14. Schwarz JM, Neese RA, Schakleton C, et al. Diabetes. 1993; 42(suppl): A39.

15. Schwarz JM, Neese RA, Turner SM, et al. Diabetes. 1994; 43(suppl): 52A.

16. Sloth B, Krog-Mikkelsen I, Flint A, et al. Am J Clin Nutr. 2004; 80: 337-47.

17. Suga A, Hirano T, Kageyama H, et al. Am J Physiol Endocrinol Metab. 2000; 278: E677-83.

18. Teff K, Elliott S, Tschoep M, et al. Diabetes. 2002; 1(suppl): 1672.

19. Teff KL, Elliott SS, Tschop M, et al. J Clin Endocrinol Metab. 2004; 89: 2963-72.

20. Wellhoener P, Fruehwald-Schultes B, Kern W, et al. J Clin Endocrinol Metab. 2000; 85: 1267-71.

Q

1. Air EL, Strowski MZ, Benoit SC, et al. Nat Med. 2002; 8: 303.

2. Benoit SC, Air EL, Coolen LM, et al. J Neurosci. 2002; 22: 9048-52.

3. Boyko EJ, Leonetti DL, Bergstrom RW, et al. Diabetes. 1996; 45: 1010-5.

4. Bruning JC, Gautam D, Burks DJ, et al. Science. 2000; 289: 2122-5.

5. Chapman IM, Goble EA, Wittert GA, et al. Am J Physiol. 1998; 274(3 Pt 2): R596-603.

6. Doucet E, Almeras N, White MD, et al. Eur J Clin Nutr. 1998; 52: 2-6.

7. Folsom AR, Vitelli LL, Lewis CE, et al. Int J Obes Relat Metab Disord. 1998; 22: 48-54.

8. Garaulet M, Marin C, Perez-Llamas F, et al. J Physiol Biochem. 2004; 60: 39-49.

9. Gazzaniga JM, Burns TL. Am J Clin Nutr. 1993; 58: 21-8.

10. Gerozissis K. Eur J Pharmacol. 2004; 490(1-3): 59-70.

11. Gerozissis K, Kyriaki G. Cell Mol Neurobiol. 2003; 23(4-5): 873-4.

12. Gerozissis K, Orosco M, Rouch C, et al. Physiol Behav. 1997; 62: 767-72.

13. Hoag S, Marshall JA, Jones RH, et al. Int J Obes Relat Metab Disord. 1995; 19: 175-80.

14. Kaiyala KJ, Prigeon RL, Kahn SE, et al. Diabetes. 2000; 49: 1525-33.

15. Lahoz C, Alonso R, Porres A, et al. Med Clin (Barc). 1999; 112: 133-7.

16. McMinn JE, Baskin DG, Schwartz MW. Obes Rev. 2000; 1: 37-46.

17. Navia B, Requejo AM, Ortega RM, et al. Ann Nutr Metab. 1997; 41: 299-306.

18. Nicklas TA, Hampl JS, Taylor CA, et al. Nutr Rev. 2004; 62: 132-41.

19. Niswender KD, Schwartz MW. Front Neuroendocrinol. 2003; 24: 1-10.

20. Obici S, Feng Z, Karkanias G, et al. Nat Neurosci. 2002; 5: 566-72.

21. Porte D Jr, Baskin DG, Schwartz MW. Nutr Rev. 2002; 60(10 Pt 2): S20-9; discussion S68-84, 85-7.

22. Porte D Jr, Woods SC. Diabetologia. 1981; 20 Suppl: 274-80.

23. Salas J, Lopez Miranda J, Jansen S, et al. Med Clin (Barc). 1999; 114: 249.

24. Schwartz MW. Exp Biol Med (Maywood). 2001; 226: 978-81.

25. Schwartz MW, Boyko EJ, Kahn SE, et al. J Clin Endocrinol Metab. 1995; 80: 1571-6.

26. Weyer C, Hanson K, Bogardus C, et al. Diabetologia. 2000; 43: 36-46.

27. Withers DJ. Biochem Soc Trans. 2001; 29(Pt 4): 525-9.

28. Woods SC, Chavez M, Park CR, et al. Neurosci Biobehav Rev. 1996; 20: 139-44.

29. Woods SC, Seeley RJ. Int J Obes Relat Metab Disord. 2001; 25 Suppl 5: S35-8.

30. Wozniak M, Rydzewski B, Baker SP, et al. Neurochem Int. 1993; 22: 1-10.

R

1. Antoine JM, Rohr R, Gagey MJ, et al. Hum Nutr Clin Nutr. 1984; 38: 31-8.

2. Arnold L, Ball M, Mann J. Atherosclerosis. 1994; 108: 167-74.

3. Arnold L, Mann JI, Ball MJ. Diabetes Care. 1997; 20: 1651-4.

4. Baker N, Huebotter RJ. J Lipid Res. 1973; 14: 87-94.

5. Baker N, Palmquist DL, Learn DB. J Lipid Res. 1976; 17: 527-35.

6. Bellisle F, McDevitt R, Prentice AM. Br J Nutr. 1997; 77 Suppl 1: S57-70.

7. Bortz W, Wroldsen A, Issekutz B, et al. N Engl J Med. 1966; 274: 376-379.

8. Bray GA. J Clin Invest. 1972; 51: 537-48.

9. Cohn C. J Am Diet Assoc. 1961; 38: 433-6.

10. Dallosso HM, Murgatroyd PR, James WP. Hum Nutr Clin Nutr. 1982; 36C(1): 25-39.

11. Finkelstein B, Fryer BA. Am J Clin Nutr. 1971; 24: 465-8.

12. Garrow JS, Durrant M, Blaza S, et al. Br J Nutr. 1981; 45: 5-15.

13. Gwinup G, Kruger FA, Hamwi GJ. Ohio State Med J. 1964; 60: 663-6.

14. Hill JO, Anderson JC, Lin D, et al. Am J Physiol. 1988; 255(4 Pt 2): R616-21.

15. Holmback U, Lowden A, Akerfeldt T, et al. J Nutr. 2003; 133: 2748-55.

16. Jenkins DJ, Wolever TM, Vuksan V, et al. N Engl J Med. 1989; 321: 929-34.

17. Jones PJ, Namchuk GL, Pederson RA. Metabolism. 1995; 44: 218-23.

18. Kinabo JL, Durnin JV. Eur J Clin Nutr. 1990; 44: 389-95.

19. LeBlanc J, Mercier I, Nadeau A. Can J Physiol Pharmacol. 1993; 71: 879-83.

20. Mann J. Br J Nutr. 1997; 77 Suppl 1: S83-90.

21. Murphy MC, Chapman C, Lovegrove JA, et al. Eur J Clin Nutr. 1996; 50: 491-7.

22. No authors listed. Nutr Rev. 1972; 30: 158-62.

23. Rashidi MR, Mahboob S, Sattarivand R. Saudi Med J. 2003; 24: 945-8.

24. Romsos DR, Miller ER, Leveille GA. Proc Soc Exp Biol Med. 1978; 157: 528-30.

25. Sensi S, Capani F. Chronobiol Int. 1987; 4: 251-61.

26. Swindells YE, Holmes SA, Robinson MF. Br J Nutr. 1968; 22: 667-680.

27. Taylor MA, Garrow JS. Int J Obes Relat Metab Disord. 2001; 25: 519-28.

28. Verboeket-van de Venne WP, Westerterp KR. Int J Obes Relat Metab Disord. 1993; 17: 31-6.

29. Verboeket-van de Venne WP, Westerterp KR. Eur J Clin Nutr. 1991; 45: 161-9.

30. Wadhwa PS, Young EA, Schmidt K, et al. Am J Clin Nutr. 1973; 26: 823-30.

31. Wolfram G, Kirchgessner M, Muller HL, et al. Ann Nutr Metab. 1987; 31: 88-97.

32. Wu H, Wu DY. Proc Soc Exp Biol Med. 1950; 74: 78-82.

33. Young CM, Hutter LF, Scanlan SS, et al. J Am Diet Assoc. 1972; 61: 391-8.

34. Young CM, Scanlan SS, Topping CM, et al. J Am Diet Assoc. 1971; 59: 466-72.

S

1. Cummings DE, Purnell JQ, Frayo RS, et al. Diabetes. 2001; 50: 1714-9.

2. Molnar D. Padiatr Padol. 1992; 27: 177-81.

3. No authors listed. Nutr Rev. 1972; 30: 158-62.

4. Tai MM, Castillo P, Pi-Sunyer FX. Am J Clin Nutr. 1991; 54: 783-7.

5. Verboeket-van de Venne WP, Westerterp KR, Kester AD. Br J Nutr. 1993; 70: 103-15.

6. Westerterp-Plantenga MS, Goris AH, Meijer EP, et al. Br J Nutr. 2003; 90: 643-9.

7. Young CM, Hutter LF, Scanlan SS, et al. J Am Diet Assoc. 1972; 61: 391-8.

8. Young CM, Scanlan SS, Topping CM, et al. J Am Diet Assoc. 1971; 59: 466-72.

9. Young JC. Eur J Appl Physiol Occup Physiol. 1995; 70: 437-41.

T

1. Avenell A, Brown TJ, McGee MA, et al. J Hum Nutr Diet. 2004; 17: 293-316.

2. Garrow JS, Summerbell CD. Eur J Clin Nutr. 1995; 49: 1-10.

3. Kirk EP, Jacobsen DJ, Gibson C, et al. Int J Obes Relat Metab Disord. 2003; 27: 912-9.

4. Pritchard JE, Nowson CA, Wark JD. J Am Diet Assoc. 1997; 97: 37-42.

U

1. Ballor DL, Poehlman ET. Int J Obes Relat Metab Disord. 1994; 18: 35-40.

2. Bryner RW, Ullrich IH, Sauers J, et al. J Am Coll Nutr. 1999; 18: 115-21.

3. Cox KL, Burke V, Morton AR, et al. Metabolism. 2003; 52: 107-15.

4. Dengel DR, Hagberg JM, Coon PJ, et al. Med Sci Sports Exerc. 1994; 26: 1307-15.

5. Dengel DR, Hagberg JM, Coon PJ, et al. Metabolism. 1994; 43: 867-71.

6. Donnelly JE, Pronk NP, Jacobsen DJ, et al. Am J Clin Nutr. 1991; 54: 56-61.

7. Donnelly JE, Sharp T, Houmard J, et al. Am J Clin Nutr. 1993; 58: 561-5.

8. Evans EM, Saunders MJ, Spano MA, et al. Am J Clin Nutr. 1999; 70: 5-12.

9. Evans EM, Saunders MJ, Spano MA, et al. Med Sci Sports Exerc. 1999; 31: 1778-87.

10. Geliebter A, Maher MM, Gerace L, et al. Am J Clin Nutr. 1997; 66: 557-63.

11. Gornall J, Villani RG. Int J Sport Nutr. 1996; 6: 285-94.

12. Janssen I, Fortier A, Hudson R, et al. Diabetes Care. 2002; 25: 431-8.

13. Klem ML, Wing RR, McGuire MT, et al. Am J Clin Nutr. 1997; 66: 239-46.

14. Kraemer WJ, Volek JS, Clark KL, et al. J Appl Physiol. 1997; 83: 270-9.

15. Lamarche B, Despres JP, Moorjani S, et al. Int J Obes Relat Metab Disord. 1993; 17: 255-61.

16. Lemons AD, Kreitzman SN, Coxon A, et al. Int J Obes. 1989; 13 Suppl 2: 119-23.

17. McGuire MT, Wing RR, Klem ML, et al. Obes Res. 1999; 7: 334-41.

18. McGuire MT, Wing RR, Klem ML, et al. Int J Obes Relat Metab Disord. 1998; 22: 572-7.

19. Nieman DC, Brock DW, Butterworth D, et al. J Am Coll Nutr. 2002; 21: 344-50.

20. Poehlman ET, Dvorak RV, DeNino WF, et al. J Clin Endocrinol Metab. 2000; 85: 2463-8.

21. Powell JJ, Tucker L, Fisher AG, et al. Am J Health Promot. 1994; 8: 442-8.

22. Schwingshandl J, Sudi K, Eibl B, et al. Arch Dis Child. 1999; 81: 426-8.

23. Stensel DJ, Brooke-Wavell K, Hardman AE, et al. Eur J Appl Physiol Occup Physiol. 1994; 68: 531-7.

24. Sweeney ME, Hill JO, Heller PA, et al. Am J Clin Nutr. 1993; 57: 127-34.

25. Utter AC, Nieman DC, Shannonhouse EM, et al. Int J Sport Nutr. 1998; 8: 213-22.

26. Van Dale D, Saris WH, Schoffelen PF, et al. Int J Obes. 1987; 11: 367-75.

A Good Start

A

1. Almdal TP, Heindorff H, Bardram L, et al. Gut. 1990; 31: 946-8.

2. Almdal TP, Vilstrup H. Endocrinology. 1988; 123: 2182-6.

3. Attvall S, Fowelin J, von Schenck H, et al. J Clin Endocrinol Metab. 1992; 74: 1110-5.

4. Benoit FL, Martin RL, Watten RH. Ann Int Med. 1965; 63: 604-612.

5. Benson JW Jr, Johnson DG, Palmer JP, et al. J Clin Endocrinol Metab. 1977; 44: 459-64.

6. Boden G, Master RW, Rezvani I, et al. J Clin Invest. 1980; 65: 706-16.

7. Boden G, Rezvani I, Owen OE. J Clin Invest. 1984; 73: 785-93.

8. Boden G, Tappy L, Jadali F, et al. Am J Physiol. 1990; 259(2 Pt 1): E225-32.

9. Brockman RP, Bergman EN. Am J Physiol. 1975; 228: 1627-33.

10. Cahill GF. Diabetes. 1971; 20: 785-99.

11. Charlton MR, Adey DB, Nair KS. J Clin Invest. 1996; 98: 90-9.

12. Charlton MR, Nair KS. Diabetes. 1998; 47: 1748-56.

13. Chhibber VL, Soriano C, Tayek JA. Metabolism. 2000; 49: 39-46.

14. Chiasson JL, Liljenquist JE, Sinclair-Smith BC, et al. Diabetes. 1975; 24: 574-84.

15. Couet C, Fukagawa NK, Matthews DE, et al. Am J Physiol. 1990; 258(1 Pt 1): E78-85.

16. Dirlewanger M, Schneiter PH, Paquot N, et al. Clin Nutr. 2000; 19: 29-34.

17. Foster GD, Wyatt HR, Hill JO, et al. N Engl J Med. 2003; 348: 2082-90.

18. Genuth SM, Hoppel CL. Metabolism. 1981; 30: 393-401.

19. Gerich JE, Lorenzi M, Bier DM, et al. N Engl J Med. 1975; 292: 985-9.

20. Guttler F, Kuhl C, Pedersen L, et al. Scand J Clin Lab Invest. 1978; 38: 255-60.

21. Hartl WH, Miyoshi H, Jahoor F, et al. Am J Physiol. 1990; 259(2 Pt 1): E239-45.

22. Jahoor F, Herndon DN, Wolfe RR. J Clin Invest. 1986; 78: 807-14.

23. Keckwick A, Pawan GL. Metabolism. 1957; 6: 447-60.

24. Lewis GF, Vranic M, Giacca A. Am J Physiol. 1997; 272(3 Pt 1): E371-8.

25. Liljenquist JE, Mueller GL, Cherrington AD, et al. J Clin Invest. 1977; 59: 369-74.

26. Liu D, Adamson U, Lins PE, et al. Diabet Med. 1993; 10: 246-54.

27. Lugari R, Maestri E, Tagliaferri A, et al. Acta Biomed Ateneo Parmense. 1981; 52(2-3): 175-80.

28. Mallinson CN, Bloom SR, Warin AP, et al. Lancet. 1974; 2: 1-5.

29. Marchini JS, Marks LM, Darmaun D, et al. Metabolism. 1998; 47: 497-502.

30. McCullough AJ, Mullen KD, Tavill AS, et al. Gastroenterology. 1992; 103: 571-8.

31. Meguid MM, Brennan MF, Aoki TT, et al. Arch Surg. 1974; 109: 776-83.

32. Nair KS. J Clin Endocrinol Metab. 1987; 64: 896-901.

33. Nair KS, Halliday D, Matthews DE, et al. Am J Physiol. 1987; 253(2 Pt 1): E208-13.

34. Ohtsuka A, Hayashi K, Noda T, et al. J Nutr Sci Vitaminol (Tokyo). 1992; 38: 83-92.

35. Phinney SD, Bistrian BR, Wolfe RR, et al. Metabolism. 1983; 32: 757-68.

36. Roth E, Mulbacher F, Karner J, et al. Metab Clin Exp. 1987; 26: 7-13.

37. Russell RCG, Walker CJ, Bloom SR. Br Med J. 1992; 1: 10-2.

38. Sherwin R, Wahren J, Felig P. Metabolism. 1976; 25(11 Suppl 1): 1381-3.

39. Soltesz G, Molnar D, Kardos M, et al. Acta Paediatr Acad Sci Hung. 1982; 23: 137-43.

40. Stevenson RW, Steiner KE, Davis MA, et al. Diabetes. 1987; 36: 382-9.

41. Surmely JF, Schneiter P, Henry S, et al. Nutrition. 1999; 15: 267-73.

42. Tessari P, Inchiostro S, Barazzoni R, et al. Diabetes. 1996; 45: 463-70.

43. Tse TF, Clutter WE, Shah SD, et al. J Clin Invest. 1983; 72: 278-86.

44. Volek JS, Sharman MJ, Love DM, et al. Metabolism. 2002; 51: 864-70.

45. Westman EC, Yancy WS, Edman JS, et al. Am J Med. 2002; 113: 30-6.

46. Wilmore DW, Molan JA, Pruitt BA, et al. Lancet. 1974; 19: 73-5.

47. Wolfe BM, Culebras JM, Aoki TT, et al. Surgery. 1979; 86: 248-57.

48. Yancy WS Jr, Olsen MK, Guyton JR, et al. Ann Intern Med. 2004; 140: 769-77.

B

1. Beylot M. Diabetes Metab. 1996; 22: 299-304.

2. Beylot M, Picard S, Chambrier C, et al. Metabolism. 1991; 40: 1138-46.

3. Boden G, Tappy L, Jadali F, et al. Am J Physiol. 1990; 259(2 Pt 1): E225-32.

4. Carlson MG, Snead WL, Campbell PJ. J Clin Endocrinol Metab. 1993; 77: 11-5.

5. Charlton MR, Adey DB, Nair KS. J Clin Invest. 1996; 98: 90-9.

6. Gerich JE, Lorenzi M, Bier DM, et al. N Engl J Med. 1975; 292: 985-9.

7. Gerich JE, Lorenzi M, Bier DM, et al. J Clin Invest. 1976; 57: 875-84.

8. Gerich JE, Schneider VS, Lorenzi M, et al. Clin Endocrinol (Oxf). 1976; 5 Suppl: 299S-305S.

9. Gill A, Johnston DG, Orskov H, et al. Metabolism. 1982; 31: 305-11.

10. Jensen MD, Heiling VJ, Miles JM. J Clin Endocrinol Metab. 1991; 72: 308-15.

11. Keller U, Schnell H, Sonnenberg GE, et al. Diabetes. 1983; 32: 387-91.

12. Kuroshima A, Doi K, Ohno T. Jpn J Physiol. 1979; 29: 661-8.

13. Merimee TJ, Misbin RI, Pulkkinen AJ. J Clin Endocrinol Metab. 1978; 46: 414-9.

14. Miles JM, Haymond MW, Gerich JE. Ciba Found Symp. 1982; 87: 192-213.

15. Miles JM, Haymond MW, Nissen SL, et al. J Clin Invest. 1983; 71: 1554-61.

16. Nair KS, Ford GC, Ekberg K, et al. J Clin Inest. 1995; 95: 2926-37.

17. Paolisso G, Buonocore S, Gentile S, et al. Diabetologia. 1990; 33: 272-7.

18. Quabbe HJ, Luyckx AS, L'age M, et al. J Clin Endocrinol Metab. 1983; 57: 410-4.

19. Roth E, Mulbacher F, Karner J, et al. Metab Clin Exp. 1987; 26: 7-13.

20. Schade DS, Eaton RP. Diabetes. 1975; 24: 502-9.

21. Schade DS, Eaton RP. Diabetes 1975; 24: 1020-6.

22. Schade DS, Eaton RP. Diabetologia. 1975; 11: 555-9.

23. Schade DS, Eaton RP. J Clin Invest. 1975; 56: 1340-4.

24. Schade DS, Eaton RP. Diabetes. 1975; 24: 510-5.

25. Schneider SH, Fineberg SE, Blackburn GL. Diabetologia. 1981; 20: 616-21.

26. Soltesz G, Molnar D, Kardos M, et al. Acta Paediatr Acad Sci Hung. 1982; 23: 137-43.

27. Sonnenberg GE, Stauffacher W, Keller U. Diabetologia. 1982; 23: 94-100.

28. Stout RW, Henry RW, Buchanan KD. Eur J Clin Invest. 1976; 6: 179-85.

29. Ubukata E, Mokuda O, Sakamoto Y, et al. Diabetes Res Clin Pract. 1996; 34: 1-6.

C

1. Fraser DA, Thoen J, Bondhus S, et al. Clin Exp Rheumatol. 2000; 18: 209-14.

2. Lewis SB, Wallin JD, Kane JP, et al. Am J Clin Nutr. 1977; 30: 160-70.

3. Volek JS, Sharman MJ, Love DM, et al. Metabolism. 2002; 51: 864-70.

D

1. Beck B, Musse N, Stricker-Krongrad A. Biochem Biophys Res Commun. 2002; 292: 1031-5.

E

1. Keckwick A, Pawan GL. Metabolism. 1957; 6: 447-60.

2. Keller U, Lustenberger M, Muller-Brand J, et al. Diabetes Metab Rev. 1989; 5: 285-98.

3. Ullrich IH, Peters PJ, Albrink MJ. J Am Coll Nutr. 1985; 4: 451-9.

4. Volek JS, Sharman MJ, Love DM, et al. Metabolism. 2002; 51: 864-70.

F

1. Ahima RS, Kelly J, Elmquist JK, et al. Endocrinology. 1999; 140: 4923-31.

2. Filozof CM, Murua C, Sanchez MP, et al. Obes Res. 2000; 8: 205-10.

3. Meister B. Vitam Horm. 2000; 59: 265-304.

4. Muzzin P, Eisensmith RC, Copeland KC, et al. Proc Natl Acad Sci U S A. 1996; 93: 14804-8.

Introducing The Carb Nite Solution

A

1. Volek JS, Sharman MJ, Love DM, et al. Metabolism. 2002; 51: 864-70.

B

1. Boisjoyeux B, Chanez M, Azzout B, et al. Diabete Metab. 1986; 12: 21-7.

2. Calbet JA, MacLean DA. J Nutr. 2002; 132: 2174-82.

3. Day JL, Johansen K, Ganda OP, et al. Clin Endocrinol (Oxf). 1978; 9: 443-54.

4. De Santo NG, Capasso G, Anastasio P, et al. Ren Physiol Biochem. 1992; 15: 53-6.

5. Eisenstein AB, Strack I, Gallo-Torres H, et al. Am J Physiol. 1979; 236: E20-7.

6. Gannon MC, Nuttall FQ, Lane JT, et al. Metabolism. 1992; 41: 1137-45.

7. Gevrey JC, Malapel M, Philippe J, et al. Diabetologia. 2004; 47: 926-36.

8. Hamberg O, Andersen V, Sonne J, et al. Clin Nutr. 2001; 20: 493-501.

9. Hubbard R, Kosch CL, Sanchez A, et al. Atherosclerosis. 1989; 76: 55-61.

10. Krebs M, Brehm A, Krssak M, et al. Diabetologia. 2003; 46: 917-25.

11. Krezowski PA, Nuttall FQ, Gannon MC, et al. Am J Clin Nutr. 1986; 44: 847-56.

12. Lang V, Bellisle F, Alamowitch C, et al. Eur J Clin Nutr. 1999; 53: 959-65.

13. LeBlanc J, Soucy J, Nadeau A. Horm Metab Res. 1996; 28: 276-9.

14. Linn T, Santosa B, Gronemeyer D, et al. Diabetologia. 2000; 43: 1257-65.

15. Matzen LE, Andersen BB, Jensen BG, et al. Scand J Clin Lab Invest. 1990; 50: 801-5.

16. Sanchez A, Hubbard RW, Smit E, et al. Atherosclerosis. 1988; 71: 87-92.

17. Schmid R, Schulte-Frohlinde E, Schusdziarra V, et al. Pancreas. 1992; 7: 698-704.

18. Schmid R, Schusdziarra V, Schulte-Frohlinde E, et al. J Clin Endocrinol Metab. 1989; 68: 1106-10.

19. Schmid R, Schusdziarra V, Schulte-Frohlinde E, et al. Pancreas. 1989; 4: 305-14.

20. Sugano M, Ishiwaki N, Nagata Y, et al. Br J Nutr. 1982; 48: 211-21.

21. Tovar AR, Ascencio C, Torres N. Am J Physiol Endocrinol Metab. 2002; 283: E1016-22.

22. Westphal SA, Gannon MC, Nuttall FQ. Am J Clin Nutr. 1990; 52: 267-72.

23. Wright PD, Holdsworth JD, Dionigi P, et al. Gut. 1986; 27 Suppl 1: 96-102.

C

1. Benoit FL, Martin RL, Watten RH. Ann Int Med. 1965; 63: 604-612.

2. Schrauwen P, van Marken Lichtenbelt WD, Saris WH, et al. Am J Clin Nutr. 1997; 66: 276-82.

D

1. Rothwell NJ, Saville ME, Stock MJ. Am J Physiol. 1982; 243: R339-46.

2. Weigle DS, Duell PB, Connor WE, et al. J Clin Endocrinol Metab. 1997; 82: 561-5.

E

1. Beulens JW, Bindels JG, de Graaf C, et al. Physiol Behav. 2004; 81: 585-93.

2. Fadda F, Cocco S, Stancampiano R. Brain Res Brain Res Protoc. 2000; 5: 219-22.

3. Fernstrom JD, Faller DV, Shabshelowitz H. J Neural Transm. 1975; 36: 113-21.

4. Fernstrom JD, Wurtman RJ, Hammarstrom-Wiklund B, et al. Am J Clin Nutr. 1979; 32: 1912-22.

5. Feurte S, Gerozissis K, Regnault A, et al. Nutr Neurosci. 2001; 4: 413-8.

6. Fischer K, Colombani PC, Langhans W, et al. Physiol Behav. 2002; 75: 411-23.

7. Kaye WH, Gwirtsman HE, Brewerton TD, et al. Psychiatry Res. 1988; 23: 31-43.

8. Leyton M, Pun VK, Benkelfat C, et al. J Psychiatry Neurosci. 2003; 28: 464-7.

9. Lieben CK, Blokland A, Westerink B, et al. Neurochem Int. 2004; 44: 9-16.

10. Markus CR, Olivier B, de Haan EH. Am J Clin Nutr. 2002; 75: 1051-6.

11. Markus CR, Olivier B, Panhuysen GE, et al. Am J Clin Nutr. 2000; 71: 1536-44.

12. Markus CR, Panhuysen G, Tuiten A, et al. Appetite. 1998; 31: 49-65.

13. Moller SE. A preliminary study. Hum Neurobiol.1983; 2: 45-8.

14. Orosco M, Rouch C, Beslot F, et al. Behav Brain Res. 2004; 148(1-2): 1-10.

15. Rouch C, Meile MJ, Orosco M. Nutr Neurosci. 2003; 6: 117-24.

16. Ruggiero M, Perna M, Morelli S, et al. Boll Soc Ital Biol Sper. 1981; 57: 2123-9.

17. Uhe AM, Collier GR, O'Dea K. J Nutr. 1992; 122: 467-72.

18. Unge G, Malmgren R, Olsson P, et al. Cephalalgia. 1983; 3: 213-8.

19. Weltzin TE, Fernstrom JD, McConaha C, et al. Biol Psychiatry. 1994; 35: 388-97.

20. Wurtman RJ, Wurtman JJ, Regan MM, et al. Am J Clin Nutr. 2003; 77: 128-32.

F

1. Boss O, Samec S, Kuhne F, et al. J Biol Chem. 1998; 273: 5-8.

2. Dallongeville J, Hecquet B, Lebel P, et al. Int J Obes Relat Metab Disord. 1998; 22: 728-33.

3. Dallosso HM, James WP. 2. 1984; 52: 65-72.

4. Danforth E Jr, Horton ES, O'Connell M, et al. J Clin Invest. 1979; 64: 1336-47.

5. Dobrohorska H, Sulima D, Oskaldowicz K, et al. Acta Physiol Pol. 1981; 32: 703-12.

6. Glick Z, Wu SY, Lupien J, et al. Am J Physiol. 1985; 249(5 Pt 1): E519-24.

7. Gong DW, He Y, Karas M, et al. J Biol Chem. 1997; 272: 24129-32.

8. Gray DS, Takahashi M, Fisler JS, et al. Metabolism. 1989; 38: 208-14.

9. Horton TJ, Drougas H, Brachey A, et al. Am J Clin Nutr. 1995; 62: 19-29.

10. Horton TJ, Hill JO. J Appl Physiol. 2001; 90: 155-63.

11. Jaedig S, Faber J. Acta Endocrinol (Copenh). 1982; 100: 388-92.

12. Jenkins AB, Markovic TP, Fleury A, et al. Diabetologia. 1997; 40: 348-51.

13. Kmiec Z, Kotlarz G, Smiechowska B, et al. J Endocrinol Invest. 1996; 19: 304-11.

14. Kolaczynski JW, Considine RV, Ohannesian J, et al. Diabetes. 1996; 45: 1511-5.

15. Kolaczynski JW, Ohannesian JP, Considine RV, et al. J Clin Endocrinol Metab. 1996; 81: 4162-5.

16. Koppeschaar HP, Meinders AE, Schwarz F. The role of sympathetic nervous system activity and thyroid hormones. 1985; 39: 17-28.

17. LoPresti JS, Gray D, Nicoloff JT. J Clin Endocrinol Metab. 1991; 72: 130-6.

18. Marques-Lopes I, Ansorena D, Astiasaran I, et al. Am J Clin Nutr. 2001; 73: 253-61.

19. Marques-Lopes I, Forga L, Martinez JA. Nutrition. 2003; 19: 25-9.

20. McDevitt RM, Poppitt SD, Murgatroyd PR, et al. Am J Clin Nutr. 2000; 72: 369-77.

21. Monteleone P, Bortolotti F, Fabrazzo M, et al. J Clin Endocrinol Metab. 2000; 85: 2499-503.

22. Pilegaard H, Saltin B, Neufer PD. Diabetes. 2003; 52: 657-62.

23. Romon M, Lebel P, Fruchart JC, et al. J Am Coll Nutr. 2003; 22: 247-51.

24. Romon M, Lebel P, Velly C, et al. Am J Physiol. 1999; 277(5 Pt 1): E855-61.

25. Rothwell NJ, Saville ME, Stock MJ. Am J Physiol. 1982; 243: R339-46.

26. Schebendach JE, Golden NH, Jacobson MS, et al. Ann N Y Acad Sci. 1997; 817: 110-9.

27. Stock MJ. Eur J Appl Physiol Occup Physiol. 1980; 43: 35-40.

28. Sugden MC, Kraus A, Harris RA, et al. Biochem J. 2000; 346 Pt 3: 651-7.

29. Taskinen MR, Nikkila EA. Metabolism. 1987; 36: 625-30.

30. Tunstall RJ, Mehan KA, Hargreaves M, et al. Biochem Biophys Res Commun. 2002; 294: 301-8.

31. Weigle DS, Duell PB, Connor WE, et al. J Clin Endocrinol Metab. 1997; 82: 561-5.

32. Weigle DS, Selfridge LE, Schwartz MW, et al. Diabetes. 1998; 47: 298-302.

33. Westerterp KR, Wilson SA, Rolland V. Int J Obes Relat Metab Disord. 1999; 23: 287-92.

34. Weyer C, Vozarova B, Ravussin E, et al. Int J Obes Relat Metab Disord. 2001; 25: 593-600.

35. Wisse BE, Campfield LA, Marliss EB, et al. Am J Clin Nutr. 1999; 70: 321-30.

36. Woods SC, Seeley RJ, Baskin DG, et al. Curr Pharm Des. 2003; 9: 795-800.

G

1. Choi YH, Li CL, Hartzell DL, et al. Domest Anim Endocrinol. 2003; 25: 295-301.

2. Commins SP, Watson PM, Frampton IC, et al. Am J Physiol Endocrinol Metab. 2001; 280: E372-7.

3. Gullicksen PS, Hausman DB, Dean RG, et al. Int J Obes Relat Metab Disord. 2003; 27: 302-12.

4. Loftus TM, Kuhajda FP, Lane MD. Proc Natl Acad Sci U S A. 1998; 95: 14168-72.

5. Qian H, Azain MJ, Compton MM, et al. Endocrinology. 1998; 139: 791-4.

H

1. Miller JC, Colagiuri S. Diabetologia. 1994; 37: 1280-6.

2. Phinney SD, Bistrian BR, Wolfe RR, et al. Metabolism. 1983; 32: 757-68.

I

1. Atwater WO, Woods CD. The availability and fuel values of food materials. In Connecticut (Storrs) Agricultural Experiment Station 12th Annual Report (Storrs, CT). 1900; 73-123.

2. Carew LB Jr, Hill FW. J Nutr. 1964; 83: 293-9.

3. Carew LB Jr, Hopkins DT, Nesheim MC. J Nutr. 1964; 83: 300-6.

4. Donato K, Hegsted DM. Proc Natl Acad Sci U S A. 1985; 82: 4866-70.

5. Donato KA. Am J Clin Nutr. 1987; 45(1 Suppl): 164-7.

A Little Word About Food

A

1. Binnert C, Pachiaudi C, Beylot M, et al. Am J Physiol. 1996; 270(3 Pt 1): E445-50.

2. Hansen JB, Grimsgaard S, Nilsen H, et al. Lipids. 1998; 33: 131-8.

3. Heath RB, Karpe F, Milne RW, et al. J Lipid Res. 2003; 44: 2065-72.

4. Yli-Jokipii K, Kallio H, Schwab U, et al. J Lipid Res. 2001; 42: 1618-25.

B

1. Aro A, Jauhiainen M, Partanen R, et al. Am J Clin Nutr. 1997; 65: 1419-26.

2. Bonanome A, Grundy SM. N Engl J Med. 1988; 318: 1244-8.

3. Brehm BJ, Seeley RJ, Daniels SR, et al. J Clin Endocrinol Metab. 2003; 88: 1617-23.

4. Denke MA, Grundy SM. Am J Clin Nutr. 1991; 54: 1036-40.

5. Dougherty RM, Allman MA, Iacono JM. Am J Clin Nutr. 1995; 61: 1120-8.

6. Foster GD, Wyatt HR, Hill JO, et al. N Engl J Med. 2003; 348: 2082-90.

7. Hayes KC. Can J Cardiol. 1995; 11 Suppl G: 39G-46G.

8. Hays JH, DiSabatino A, Gorman RT, et al. Mayo Clin Proc. 2003; 78: 1331-6.

9. Hu FB, Stampfer MJ, Manson JE, et al. Am J Clin Nutr. 1999; 70: 1001-8.

10. Judd JT, Baer DJ, Clevidence BA, et al. Lipids. 2002; 37: 123-31.

11. Kelly FD, Sinclair AJ, Mann NJ, et al. Eur J Clin Nutr. 2001; 55: 88-96.

12. Kris-Etherton PM, Mustad VA. Am J Clin Nutr. 1994; 60(6 Suppl): 1029S-1036S.

13. Lewis SB, Wallin JD, Kane JP, et al. Am J Clin Nutr. 1977; 30: 160-70.

14. Louheranta AM, Turpeinen AK, Schwab US, et al. Metabolism. 1998; 47: 529-34.

15. Meckling KA, Gauthier M, Grubb R, et al. Can J Physiol Pharmacol. 2002; 80: 1095-105.

16. Meckling KA, O'Sullivan C, Saari D. J Clin Endocrinol Metab. 2004; 89: 2717-23.

17. Rabast U, Kasper H, Schonborn J. Nutr Metab. 1978; 22: 269-77.

18. Rabast U, Vornberger KH, Ehl M. Ann Nutr Metab. 1981; 25: 341-9.

19. Salter AM, Mangiapane EH, Bennett AJ, et al. Br J Nutr. 1998; 79: 195-202.

20. Samaha FF, Iqbal N, Seshadri P, et al. N Engl J Med. 2003; 348: 2074-81.

21. Schwab US, Maliranta HM, Sarkkinen ES, et al. Metabolism. 1996; 45: 143-9.

22. Sharman MJ, Gomez AL, Kraemer WJ, et al. J Nutr. 2004; 134: 880-5.

23. Sharman MJ, Volek JS. Clin Sci (Lond). 2004; 107: 365-9.

24. Snook JT, Park S, Williams G, et al. Eur J Clin Nutr. 1999; 53: 597-605.

25. Sondike SB, Copperman N, Jacobson MS. J Pediatr. 2003; 142: 253-8.

26. Stern L, Iqbal N, Seshadri P, et al. Ann Intern Med. 2004; 140: 778-85.

27. Storm H, Thomsen C, Pedersen E, et al. Diabetes Care. 1997; 20: 1807-13.

28. Tholstrup T, Marckmann P, Jespersen J, et al. Am J Clin Nutr. 1994; 59: 371-7.

29. Thompson PD, Cullinane EM, Eshleman R, et al. Metabolism. 1984; 33: 1003-10.

30. Volek JS, Sharman MJ, Gomez AL, et al. J Am Coll Nutr. 2004; 23: 177-84.

31. Westman EC, Yancy WS, Edman JS, et al. Am J Med. 2002; 113: 30-6.

32. Yancy WS Jr, Olsen MK, Guyton JR, et al. Ann Intern Med. 2004; 140: 769-77.

33. Yu S, Derr J, Etherton TD, et al. Am J Clin Nutr. 1995; 61: 1129-39.

C

1. Doucet E, Almeras N, White MD, et al. Eur J Clin Nutr. 1998; 52: 2-6.

2. Dulloo AG, Mensi N, Seydoux J, et al. Metabolism. 1995; 44: 273-9.

3. Garaulet M, Marin C, Perez-Llamas F, et al. J Physiol Biochem. 2004; 60: 39-49.

4. Garland M, Sacks FM, Colditz GA, et al. Am J Clin Nutr. 1998; 67: 25-30.

5. Gazzaniga JM, Burns TL. Am J Clin Nutr. 1993; 58: 21-8.

6. Lahoz C, Alonso R, Porres A, et al. Med Clin (Barc). 1999; 112: 133-7.

7. London SJ, Sacks FM, Caesar J, et al. Am J Clin Nutr. 1991; 54: 340-5.

8. Lovejoy JC, Smith SR, Champagne CM, et al. Diabetes Care. 2002; 25: 1283-8.

9. Navia B, Requejo AM, Ortega RM, et al. Ann Nutr Metab. 1997; 41: 299-306.

10. Nicklas TA, Hampl JS, Taylor CA, et al. Nutr Rev. 2004; 62: 132-41.

11. Pan DA, Storlien LH. J Nutr. 1993; 123: 512-9.

12. Raclot T, Oudart H. Biochem J. 2000; 348 Pt 1: 129-36.

13. Salas J, Lopez Miranda J, Jansen S, et al. Med Clin (Barc). 1999; 114: 249.

14. Summers LK, Barnes SC, Fielding BA, et al. Am J Clin Nutr. 2000; 71: 1470-7.

15. van Staveren WA, Deurenberg P, Katan MB, et al. Am J Epidemiol. 1986; 123: 455-63.

D

1. Burdge GC, Wootton SA. Prostaglandins Leukot Essent Fatty Acids. 2003; 69: 283-90.

2. Dunham WR, Klein SB, Rhodes LM, et al. J Invest Dermatol. 1996; 107: 332-5.

3. Eaton SB, Konner M. N Engl J Med. 1985; 312: 283-9.

4. Fickova M, Hubert P, Cremel G, et al. J Nutr. 1998; 128: 512-9.

5. Ge Y, Chen Z, Kang ZB, et al. Anticancer Res. 2002; 22(2A): 537-43.

6. Kromhout D. Med Oncol Tumor Pharmacother. 1990; 7(2-3): 173-6.

7. Laidlaw M, Holub BJ. Am J Clin Nutr. 2003; 77: 37-42.

8. Lund EK, Harvey LJ, Ladha S, et al. Ann Nutr Metab. 1999; 43: 290-300.

9. Maillard V, Bougnoux P, Ferrari P, et al. Int J Cancer. 2002; 98: 78-83.

10. Okita M, Yoshida S, Yamamoto J, et al. J Nutr Sci Vitaminol (Tokyo). 1995; 41: 313-23.

11. Okuyama H, Kobayashi T, Watanabe S. Prog Lipid Res. 1996; 35: 409-57.

12. Raheja BS, Sadikot SM, Phatak RB, et al. Ann N Y Acad Sci. 1993; 683: 258-71.

13. Simopoulos AP. Poult Sci. 2000; 79: 961-70.

14. Stillwell W, Wassall SR. Chem Phys Lipids. 2003; 126: 1-27.

15. Watkins BA, Li Y, Allen KG, et al. J Nutr. 2000; 130: 2274-84.

16. Wijendran V, Hayes KC. Annu Rev Nutr. 2004; 24: 597-615.

E

1. Adlof RO, Duval S, Emken EA. Lipids. 2000; 35: 131-5.

2. Badami RC, Patil KB. Prog Lipid Res. 1981; 19: 119–53.

3. De Greyt W, Radanyi O, Kellens M, et al. Eur J Med Res. 1995; 1: 105-8.

4. Elias SL, Innis SM. J Am Diet Assoc. 2002; 102: 46-51.

5. Emken EA. Annu Rev Nutr. 1984; 4: 339-76.

6. Enig MG, Atal S, Keeney M, et al. S. 1990; 10: 514.

7. French P, Stanton C, Lawless F, et al. J Anim Sci. 2000; 78: 2849-55.

8. Henninger M, Ulberth F. Z Lebensm Unters Forsch. 1996; 203: 210-5.

9. Iwabuchi M, Kohno-Murase J, Imamura J. J Biol Chem. 2003; 278: 4603-10.

10. Jiang J, Wolk A, Vessby B. Am J Clin Nutr. 1999; 70: 21-7.

11. Mir PS, McAllister TA, Scott S, et al. Am J Clin Nutr. 2004; 79(6 Suppl): 1207S-1211S.

12. No authors listed. FDA Consum. 2003; 37: 20-6.

13. Smith CR. Prog Chem Fats Other Lipids. 1971; 11: 137–77.

F

1. Chen ZY, Ratnayake WM, Fortier L, et al. Can J Physiol Pharmacol. 1995; 73: 718-23.

2. Clifton PM, Keogh JB, Noakes M. J Nutr. 2004; 134: 1848.

3. de Roos NM, Schouten EG, Katan MB. Eur J Med Res. 2003; 8: 355-7.

4. Emken EA, Rohwedder WK, Adlof RO, et al. Lipids. 1987; 22: 495-504.

5. Emken EA, Rohwedder WK, Dutton HJ, et al. Lipids. 1979; 14: 547-54.

6. Ide T, Sugano M. Biochim Biophys Acta. 1984; 794: 281-91.

7. Lemaitre RN, King IB, Patterson RE, et al. Am J Epidemiol. 1998; 148: 1085-93.

8. London SJ, Sacks FM, Caesar J, et al. Am J Clin Nutr. 1991; 54: 340-5.

9. Seppanen-Laakso T, Laakso I, Backlund P, et al. J Chromatogr B Biomed Appl. 1996; 687: 371-8.

G

1. Jablonski E, Adamska E. Vopr Pitan. 1984; (3): 38-41.

2. Jablonski E, Rafalski H. Br J Nutr. 1984; 51: 235-43.

3. Nissen S, Haymond MW. Am J Physiol. 1986; 250(6 Pt 1): E695-701.

4. Rafalski H, Jablonski E, Switoniak T. Br J Nutr. 1978; 39: 13-8.

H

1. Baglieri A, Mahe S, Benamouzig R, et al. J Nutr. 1995; 125: 1894-903.

2. Bos C, Mahe S, Gaudichon C, et al. Br J Nutr. 1999; 81: 221-6.

3. Bos C, Metges CC, Gaudichon C, et al. J Nutr. 2003; 133: 1308-15.

4. Darcy-Vrillon B, Souffrant WB, Laplace JP, et al. Reprod Nutr Dev. 1991; 31: 561-73.

5. Deutz NEP, Soeters PB. Nutr News. 1995; 143: 133-8.

6. Fouillet H, Mariotti F, Gaudichon C, et al. J Nutr. 2002; 132: 125-33.

7. Gaudichon C, Bos C, Morens C, et al. Gastroenterology. 2002; 123: 50-9.

8. Lopez de Romana G, Graham GG, Mellits ED, et al. J Nutr. 1980; 110: 1849-57.

9. Mariotti F, Mahe S, Benamouzig R, et al. J Nutr. 1999; 129: 1992-7.

10. Morens C, Bos C, Pueyo ME, et al. J Nutr. 2003; 133: 2733-40.

11. Nielsen K, Kondrup J, Elsner P, et al. Br J Nutr. 1994; 72: 69–81.

12. Pannemans DL, Wagenmakers AJ, Westerterp KR, et al. Am J Clin Nutr. 1998; 68: 1228-35.

13. Rutherfurd SM, Moughan PJ. J Dairy Sci. 1998; 81: 909-17.

I

1. Abdel-Aziz S, Hussein L, Esmail S, et al. Int J Food Sci Nutr. 1997; 48: 51-6.

2. Baker EC, Rackis JJ. Adv Exp Med Biol. 1986; 199: 349-55.

3. Balmir F, Staack R, Jeffrey E, et al. J Nutr. 1996; 126: 3046-53.

4. Barth CA, Lunding B, Schmitz M, et al. J Nutr. 1993; 123: 2195-200.

5. Caine WR, Sauer WC, Verstegen MW, et al. J Nutr. 1998; 128: 598-605.

6. Chang HC, Doerge DR. Toxicol Appl Pharmacol. 2000; 168: 244-52.

7. Doerge DR, Chang HC. J Chromatogr B Analyt Technol Biomed Life Sci. 2002; 777(1-2): 269-79.

8. Fouillet H, Mariotti F, Gaudichon C, et al. J Nutr. 2002; 132: 125-33.

9. Jabbar MA, Larrea J, Shaw RA. J Am Coll Nutr. 1997; 16: 280-2.

10. Kandulska K, Nogowski L, Szkudelski T. Reprod Nutr Dev. 1999; 39: 497-501.

11. Klein M, Schadereit R, Kuchenmeister U. Arch Tierernahr. 2000; 53: 99-125.

12. Miyagi Y, Shinjo S, Nishida R, et al. J Nutr Sci Vitaminol (Tokyo). 1997; 43: 575-80.

13. Szkudelska K, Nogowski L, Szkudelski T. J Steroid Biochem Mol Biol. 2000; 75(4-5): 265-71.

14. Szkudelska K, Szkudelski T, Nogowski L. Phytomedicine. 2002; 9: 338-45.

The Carb Nite Solution

15. Watanabe S, Terashima K, Sato Y, et al. Biofactors. 2000; 12(1-4): 233-41.

J

1. Anema SG. J Agric Food Chem. 2000; 48: 4168-75.

2. Anema SG, Li Y. J Dairy Res. 2003; 70: 73-83.

3. Anema SG, Li Y. J Agric Food Chem. 2003; 51: 1640-6.

4. Bos C, Gaudichon C, Tome D. J Am Coll Nutr. 2000; 19(2 Suppl): 191S-205S.

5. Carbonaro M, Lucarini M, Di Lullo G. Nahrung. 2000; 44: 422-5.

6. Enomoto A, Konishi M, Hachimura S, et al. Clin Immunol Immunopathol. 1993; 66: 136-42.

7. Guy EJ, Vettel HE, Pallansch MJ. J Dairy Sci. 1967; 50: 828-32.

8. Havea P, Singh H, Creamer LK. J Dairy Res. 2001; 68: 483-97.

9. Hidalgo J, Gamper E. J Dairy Sci. 1977; 60: 1515-8.

10. Ikeda S, Morris VJ. Biomacromolecules. 2002; 3: 382-9.

11. Jeanson S, Dupont D, Grattard N, et al. J Agric Food Chem. 1999; 47: 2249-54.

12. Kessler HG, Beyer HJ. Int J Biol Macromol. 1991; 13: 165-73.

13. Kilshaw PJ, Heppell LM, Ford JE. Arch Dis Child. 1982; 57: 842-7.

14. Law AJ, Leaver J. J Agric Food Chem. 2000; 48: 672-9.

15. Leonil J, Molle D, Fauquant J, et al. J Dairy Sci. 1997; 80: 2270-81.

16. Needs EC, Capellas M, Bland AP, et al. J Dairy Res. 2000; 67: 329-48.

17. Regester GO, Pearce RJ, Lee VW, et al. J Dairy Res. 1992; 59: 527-32.

18. Schorsch BC, Wilkins DK, Jonest MG, et al. J Dairy Res. 2001; 68: 471-81.

K

1. Boirie Y, Dangin M, Gachon P, et al. Proc Natl Acad Sci U S A. 1997; 94: 14930-5.

2. Boirie Y, Gachon P, Beaufrere B. Am J Clin Nutr. 1997; 65: 489-95.

3. Boirie Y, Gachon P, Corny S, et al. Am J Physiol. 1996; 271(6 Pt 1): E1083-91.

4. Dangin M, Boirie Y, Garcia-Rodenas C, et al. Am J Physiol Endocrinol Metab. 2001; 280: E340-8.

5. Dangin M, Boirie Y, Guillet C, et al. J Nutr. 2002; 132: 3228S-33S.

6. Dangin M, Guillet C, Garcia-Rodenas C, et al. J Physiol. 2003; 549(Pt 2): 635-44.

7. Hall WL, Millward DJ, Long SJ, et al. Br J Nutr. 2003; 89: 239-48.

8. Pantako OT, Amiot J. Reprod Nutr Dev. 2001; 41: 227-38.

L

1. Bartfay WJ, Davis MT, Medves JM, et al. Can J Cardiol. 2003; 19: 1163-8.

2. Baruchel S, Viau G. Anticancer Res. 1996; 16(3A): 1095-9.

3. Bounous G. Anticancer Res. 2000; 20(6C): 4785-92.

4. Bounous G, Baruchel S, Falutz J, et al. Clin Invest Med. 1993; 16: 204-9.

5. Bounous G, Batist G, Gold P. Clin Invest Med. 1989; 12: 154-61.

6. Bounous G, Gervais F, Amer V, et al. Clin Invest Med. 1989; 12: 343-9.

7. Bounous G, Gold P. Clin Invest Med. 1991; 14: 296-309.

8. Bounous G, Molson JH. Anticancer Res. 2003; 23(2B): 1411-5.

9. Boya P, de la Pena A, Beloqui O, et al. J Hepatol. 1999; 31: 808-14.

10. de Quay B, Malinverni R, Lauterburg BH. AIDS. 1992; 6: 815-9.

11. Dickinson DA, Forman HJ. Ann N Y Acad Sci. 2002; 973: 488-504.

12. Dringen R, Hirrlinger J. Biol Chem. 2003; 384: 505-16.

13. Erden-Inal M, Sunal E, Kanbak G. Cell Biochem Funct. 2002; 20: 61-6.

14. Exner R, Wessner B, Manhart N, et al. Wien Klin Wochenschr. 2000; 112: 610-6.

15. Glosli H, Tronstad KJ, Wergedal H, et al. FASEB J. 2002; 16: 1450-2.

16. Habif S, Mutaf I, Turgan N, et al. Clin Biochem. 2001; 34: 667-71.

17. Hassan MQ, Hadi RA, Al-Rawi ZS, et al. J Appl Toxicol. 2001; 21: 69-73.

18. Kent KD, Harper WJ, Bomser JA. Toxicol In Vitro. 2003; 17: 27-33.

19. Lee YY, Kim HG, Jung HI, et al. Mol Cells. 2002; 14: 305-11.

20. Lusini L, Tripodi SA, Rossi R, et al. Int J Cancer. 2001; 91: 55-9.

21. Lyons J, Rauh-Pfeiffer A, Yu YM, et al. Proc Natl Acad Sci U S A. 2000; 97: 5071-6.

22. Mariotti F, Simbelie KL, Makarios-Lahham L, et al. J Nutr. 2004; 134: 128-31.

23. Marshall K. Altern Med Rev. 2004; 9: 136-156.

24. Matsubara LS, Machado PE. Braz J Med Biol Res. 1991; 24: 449-54.

25. Micke P, Beeh KM, Buhl R. Eur J Nutr. 2002; 41: 12-8.

26. Micke P, Beeh KM, Schlaak JF, et al. Eur J Clin Invest. 2001; 31: 171-8.

27. Mickisch G, Bier H, Bergler W, et al. Urol Int. 1990; 45: 170-6.

28. Middleton N, Jelen P, Bell G. Int J Food Sci Nutr. 2004; 55: 131-41.

29. Mytilineou C, Kramer BC, Yabut JA. Parkinsonism Relat Disord. 2002; 8: 385-7.

30. Navarro J, Obrador E, Carretero J, et al. Free Radic Biol Med. 1999; 26(3-4): 410-8.

31. Navarro J, Obrador E, Pellicer JA, et al. Free Radic Biol Med. 1997; 22: 1203-9.

32. Palomero J, Galan AI, Munoz ME, et al. Changes in liver glutathione and antioxidant enzymes. 2001; 30: 836-45.

33. Peng X, Li Y. Pharmacol Res. 2002; 45: 491-7.

34. Perego P, Paolicchi A, Tongiani R, et al. Int J Cancer. 1997; 71: 246-50.

35. Rahman I, MacNee W. Eur Respir J. 2000; 16: 534-54.

36. Rahman Q, Abidi P, Afaq F, et al. Crit Rev Toxicol. 1999; 29: 543-68.

37. Rana SV, Allen T, Singh R. Indian J Exp Biol. 2002; 40: 706-16.

38. Saralakumari D, Rao PR. Biochem Int. 1991; 23: 349-57.

39. Sido B, Hack V, Hochlehnert A, et al. Gut. 1998; 42: 485-92.

40. Stella V, Postaire E. C R Seances Soc Biol Fil. 1995; 189: 1191-7.

41. Townsend DM, Tew KD, Tapiero H. Biomed Pharmacother. 2003; 57(3-4): 145-55.

42. Wernerman J, Luo JL, Hammarqvist F. Proc Nutr Soc. 1999; 58: 677-80.

M

1. Dahlquist G, Persson B. Pediatr Res. 1976; 10: 910-7.

2. DeVivo DC, Leckie MP, Ferrendelli JS, et al. Ann Neurol. 1978; 3: 331-37.

3. Edmond J, Robbins RA, Bergstrom JD, et al. J Neurosci Res. 1987; 18: 551-61.

4. Fery F, Bourdoux P, Christophe J, et al. Diabete Metab. 1982; 8: 299-305.

5. Hasselbalch SG, Knudsen GM, Jakobsen J, et al. J Cereb Blood Flow Metab. 1994; 14: 125-31.

6. Hawkins RA, Biebuyck JF. Science. 1979; 205: 325-7.

7. Haymond MW, Howard C, Ben-Galim E, et al. Am J Physiol. 1983; 245: E373-8.

8. Mitchell GA, Kassovska-Bratinova S, Boukaftane Y, et al. Clin Invest Med. 1995; 18: 193-216.

9. Nehlig A. Prostaglandins Leukot Essent Fatty Acids. 2004; 70: 265-75.

10. Owen OE, Morgan AP, Kemp HG, et al. J Clin Invest. 1967; 46: 1589-95.

11. Pan JW, de Graaf RA, Petersen KF, et al. J Cereb Blood Flow Metab. 2002; 22: 890-8.

12. Yeh YY, Sheehan PM. Fed Proc. 1985; 44: 2352-8.

13. Yudkoff M, Daikhin Y, Nissim I, et al. J Neurosci Res. 2001; 66: 272-81.

N

1. Asp NG. Am J Clin Nutr. 1995; 61(4 Suppl): 930S-937S.

2. Behall KM, Howe JC. Am J Clin Nutr. 1995; 62(5 Suppl): 1158S-1160S.

3. Beyer-Sehlmeyer G, Glei M, Hartmann E, et al. Br J Nutr. 2003; 90: 1057-70.

4. Bourquin LD, Titgemeyer EC, Fahey GC Jr. J Nutr. 1993; 123: 860-9.

5. Bourquin LD, Titgemeyer EC, Fahey GC Jr, et al. Scand J Gastroenterol. 1993; 28: 249-55.

6. Bourquin LD, Titgemeyer EC, Garleb KA, et al. J Nutr. 1992; 122: 1508-20.

7. Cummings JH, Beatty ER, Kingman SM, et al. Br J Nutr. 1996; 75: 733-47.

8. Daniel M, Wisker E, Rave G, et al. J Nutr. 1997; 127: 1981-8.

9. Dongowski G, Lorenz A, Anger H. Appl Environ Microbiol. 2000; 66: 1321-7.

10. Ehle FR, Robertson JB, Van Soest PJ. J Nutr. 1982; 112: 158-66.

11. Ferguson LR, Tasman-Jones C, Englyst H, et al. Nutr Cancer. 2000; 36: 230-7.

12. Fernandes J, Rao AV, Wolever TM. J Nutr. 2000; 130: 1932-6.

13. Fleming SE, Rodriguez MA. J Nutr. 1983; 113: 1613-25.

14. Friedel D, Levine GM. JPEN J Parenter Enteral Nutr. 1992; 16: 1-4.

15. Hara H, Haga S, Kasai T, et al. J Nutr. 1998; 128: 688-93.

16. Jenkins DJ, Kendall CW, Vuksan V, et al. J Am Coll Nutr. 1999; 18: 339-45.

17. Kishimoto Y, Wakabayashi S, Takeda H. J Nutr Sci Vitaminol (Tokyo). 1995; 41: 151-61.

18. Kleessen B, Stoof G, Proll J, et al. J Anim Sci. 1997; 75: 2453-62.

19. Le Leu RK, Brown IL, Hu Y, et al. Carcinogenesis. 2003; 24: 1347-52.

20. Macfarlane GT, Gibson GR, Cummings JH. J Appl Bacteriol. 1992; 72: 57-64.

21. Miller TL, Wolin MJ. Appl Environ Microbiol. 1981; 42: 400-7.

22. Mortensen PB, Holtug K, Rasmussen HS. J Nutr. 1988; 118: 321-5.

23. Muir JG, Lu ZX, Young GP, et al. Am J Clin Nutr. 1995; 61: 792-9.

24. Nordgaard I, Mortensen PB, Langkilde AM. Nutrition. 1995; 11: 129-37.

25. Olesen M, Rumessen JJ, Gudmand-Hoyer E. Eur J Clin Nutr. 1994; 48: 692-701.

26. Prosky L. J AOAC Int. 2000; 83: 985-7.

27. Prosky L. J AOAC Int. 1999; 82: 223-6.

28. Ross AH, Eastwood MA, Brydon WG, et al. Am J Clin Nutr. 1983; 37: 368-75.

29. Salvador V, Cherbut C, Barry JL, et al. Br J Nutr. 1993; 70: 189-97.

30. Siragusa RJ, Cerda JJ, Baig MM, et al. Am J Clin Nutr. 1988; 47: 848-51.

31. Stark AH, Madar Z. J Nutr. 1993; 123: 2166-73.

32. Stephen AM. Crit Rev Food Sci Nutr. 1994; 34(5-6): 499-511.

33. Sunvold GD, Hussein HS, Fahey GC Jr, et al. J Anim Sci. 1995; 73: 3639-48.

34. Titgemeyer EC, Bourquin LD, Fahey GC Jr, et al. Am J Clin Nutr. 1991; 53: 1418-24.

35. Tomlin J, Read NW. Br J Nutr. 1988; 60: 467-75.

36. Topping DL, Clifton PM. Physiol Rev. 2001; 81: 1031-64.

37. Trowell H. Am J Clin Nutr. 1978; 31(10 Suppl): S3-S11.

38. van Munster IP, Tangerman A, Nagengast FM. Dig Dis Sci. 1994; 39: 834-42.

39. Wisker E, Daniel M, Rave G, et al. Br J Nutr. 2000; 84: 31-7.

40. Younes H, Coudray C, Bellanger J, et al. Br J Nutr. 2001; 86: 479-85.

41. Younes H, Levrat MA, Demigne C, et al. Ann Nutr Metab. 1993; 37: 311-9.

O

1. Miller WC, Niederpruem MG, Wallace JP, et al. J Am Diet Assoc. 1994; 94: 612-5.

2. Nelson LH, Tucker LA. J Am Diet Assoc. 1996; 96: 771-7.

P

1. Akgun S, Ertel NH. Diabetes Care. 1980; 3: 582-5.

2. Akgun S, Ertel NH. Diabetes Care. 1985; 8: 279-83.

3. Anderson JW, Story LJ, Zettwoch NC, et al. Diabetes Care. 1989; 12: 337-44.

4. Baker N, Learn DB, Bruckdorfer KR. J Lipid Res. 1978; 19: 879-93.

5. Bakr AA. Nahrung. 1997; 41: 170-5.

6. Bantle JP, Swanson JE, Thomas W, et al. Diabetes Care. 1992; 15: 1468-76.

7. Berg G, Matzkies F, Heid H, et al. Z Ernahrungswiss. 1975; 14: 163-74.

8. Carmona A, Freedland RA. J Nutr. 1989; 119: 1304-10.

9. Crapo PA, Kolterman OG, Olefsky JM. Diabetes Care. 1980; 3: 575-82.

10. Crapo PA, Scarlett JA, Kolterman OG. Am J Clin Nutr. 1982; 36: 256-61.

11. Curry DL. Pancreas. 1989; 4: 2-9.

12. de Kalbermatten N, Ravussin E, Maeder E, et al. Metabolism. 1980; 29: 62-7.

13. Elliott SS, Keim NL, Stern JS, et al. Am J Clin Nutr. 2002; 76: 911-22.

14. Frtel NH, Akgun S, Kemp FW, et al. J Nutr. 1983; 113: 566-73.

15. Fiebig R, Griffiths MA, Gore MT, et al. J Nutr. 1998; 128: 810-7.

16. Forster H. Infusionsther Klin Ernahr. 1975; 2: 187-201.

17. Forster H. Infusionsther Klin Ernahr. 1987; 14: 98-109.

18. Forster H. Int Z Vitam Ernahrungsforsch Beih. 1976; 15: 116-30.

19. Forster H, Boecker S, Walther A. Fortschr Med. 1977; 95; 99-102.

20. Forster H, Boecker S, Zagel D. Z Ernahrungswiss. 1978; 17: 224-39.

21. Forster H, Quadbeck R, Gottstein U. Int J Vitam Nutr Res Suppl. 1982; 22: 67-88.

22. Fritz M, Siebert G, Kasper H. Br J Nutr. 1985; 54: 389-400.

23. Ganda OP, Soeldner JS, Gleason RE, et al. J Clin Endocrinol Metab. 1979; 49: 616-22.

24. Gleeson M, Maughan RJ, Greenhaff PL. Eur J Appl Physiol Occup Physiol. 1986; 55: 645-53.

25. Grant AM, Christie MR, Ashcroft SJ. Diabetologia. 1980; 19: 114-7.

26. Griffiths MA, Baker DH, Novakofski JE, et al. J Am Coll Nutr. 1993; 12: 155-61.

27. Halperin ML, Cheema-Dhadli S. Biochem J. 1982; 202: 717-21.

28. Hamberg O, Almdal TP. JPEN J Parenter Enteral Nutr. 1996; 20: 139-44.

29. Hara E, Saito M. Endocrinology. 1981; 109: 966-70.

30. Hassinger W, Sauer G, Cordes U, et al. Diabetologia. 1981; 21: 37-40.

31. Havel PJ. Exp Clin Endocrinol Diabetes. 1997; 105: 37-38.

32. Havel PJ, Elliot SS, Tschoep M, et al. J Invest Med. 2002; 50: 26A (abstract).

33. Herfarth H, Klingebiel L, Juhr NC, et al. Z Ernahrungswiss. 1994; 33: 185-94.

34. Herzberg GR, Rogerson M. Br J Nutr. 1988; 59: 233-41.

35. Huttunen JK. Int Z Vitam Ernahrungsforsch Beih. 1976; 15: 105-15.

36. Ishikawa M, Miyashita M, Kawashima Y, et al. Regul Toxicol Pharmacol. 1996; 24(2 Pt 2): S303-8.

37. Jijakli H, Malaisse WJ. Acta Diabetol. 2000; 37: 27-32.

38. Kanarek RB, Orthen-Gambill N. J Nutr. 1982; 112: 1546-54.

39. Kasim-Karakas SE, Vriend H, Almario R, et al. J Lab Clin Med. 1996; 128: 208-13.

40. Kaspar L, Irsigler K. Wien Klin Wochenschr. 1980; 92: 683-7.

41. Kawai K, Okuda Y, Yamashita K. Endocrinol Jpn. 1985; 32: 933-6.

42. Kazumi T, Vranic M, Steiner G. Am J Physiol. 1986; 250(3 Pt 1): E325-30.

43. Kazumi T, Yoshino G, Matsuba K, et al. Metabolism. 1991; 40: 962-6.

44. Kuczmarski RJ, Flegal KM, Campbell SM, et al. JAMA. 1994; 272: 205-11.

45. Langkilde AM, Andersson H, Schweizer TF, et al. A study in ileostomy subjects. 1994; 48: 768-75.

46. Lee BM, Wolever TM. Eur J Clin Nutr. 1998; 52: 924-8.

47. Lian-Loh R, Birch GG, Coates ME. Br J Nutr. 1982; 48: 477-81.

48. Makinen KK. Swed Dent J. 1984; 8: 113-24.

49. Maughan RJ, Gleeson M. Eur J Appl Physiol Occup Physiol. 1988; 57: 570-6.

50. Mehnert H. Int Z Vitam Ernahrungsforsch Beih. 1976; 15: 295-324.

51. Natah SS, Hussien KR, Tuominen JA, et al. Am J Clin Nutr. 1997; 65: 947-50.

52. Nguyen NU, Dumoulin G, Henriet MT, et al. J Clin Endocrinol Metab. 1993; 77: 388-92.

53. Nicolaiew N, Cavallero E, Gandjini H, et al. Ann Nutr Metab. 1995; 39: 71-84.

54. Nilsson U, Jagerstad M. Br J Nutr. 1987; 58: 199-206.

55. No authors listed. Pediatrics. 2004; 113(1 Pt 1): 152-4.

56. Noda K, Nakayama K, Oku T. Eur J Clin Nutr. 1994; 48: 286-92.

57. Nuttall FQ, Khan MA, Gannon MC. Metabolism. 2000; 49: 1565-71.

58. Olefsky JM, Crapo P. Diabetes Care. 1980; 3: 390-3.

59. Ostashevskaia MI, Afanas'eva NB, Valuiskova RP, et al. Vopr Pitan. 1987; (2): 23-6.

60. Otto C, Sonnichsen AC, Ritter MM, et al. Clin Investig. 1993; 71: 290-3.

61. Pellaton M, Acheson K, Maeder E, et al. JPEN J Parenter Enteral Nutr. 1978; 2: 627-33.

62. Pelletier X, Hanesse B, Bornet F, et al. Diabete Metab. 1994; 20: 291-6.

63. Petzoldt R, Lauer P, Spengler M, et al. Dtsch Med Wochenschr. 1982; 107: 1910-3.

64. Rawat AK, Menahan LA. Diabetes. 1975; 24: 926-32.

65. Rizkalla SW, Boillot J, Tricottet V, et al. Br J Nutr. 1993; 70: 199-209.

66. Rizkalla SW, Luo J, Guilhem I, et al. Mol Cell Biochem. 1992; 109: 127-32.

67. Rodin J. Appetite. 1991; 17: 213-9.

68. Rosario P, Medina JM. I. 1980; 36: 439-4.

69. Salminen S, Salminen E, Marks V. Diabetologia. 1982; 22: 480-2.

70. Schulze MB, Manson JE, Ludwig DS, et al. JAMA. 2004; 292: 927-934.

71. Schwarz JM, Neese RA, Basinger A, et al. FASEB J. 1993; 7: A867.

72. Secchi A, Pontiroli AE, Cammelli L, et al. Klin Wochenschr. 1986; 64: 265-9.

73. Sener A, Malaisse WJ. Arch Biochem Biophys. 1988; 261: 16-26.

74. Sharafetdinov KhKh, Gapparov MM, Plotnikova OA, et al. Vopr Pitan. 2002; 71: 19-23.

75. Sharafetdinov KhKh, Meshcheriakova VA, Plotnikova OA, et al. Vopr Pitan. 2002; 71: 22-6.

76. Siebert G, Grupp U. Dtsch Zahnarztl Z. 1977; 32(5 Suppl 1): S36-42.

77. Steele R, Winkler B, Altszuler N. Am J Physiol. 1971; 221: 883-8.

78. Suga A, Hirano T, Kageyama H, et al. Am J Physiol Endocrinol Metab. 2000; 278: E677-83.

79. Sugawa-Katayama Y, Morita N. J Nutr. 1977; 107: 534-8.

80. Talke H, Maier KP. Infusionstherapie. 1973; 1: 49-56.

81. Teff K, Elliott S, Tschoep M, et al. Diabetes. 2002; 1(suppl): 1672.

82. Teff KL, Elliott SS, Tschop M, et al. J Clin Endocrinol Metab. 2004; 89: 2963-72.

83. Thiebaud D, Jacot E, Schmitz H, et al. Metabolism. 1984; 33: 808-13.

84. Tobey TA, Mondon CE, Zavaroni I, et al. Metabolism. 1982; 31: 608-12.

85. Todorova S, Veleva N, Arnaudov I, et al. Vutr Boles. 1982; 21: 88-96.

86. Trimmer JK, Casazza GA, Horning MA, et al. Am J Physiol Endocrinol Metab. 2001; 280: E657-68.

87. Vaaler S, Bjorneklett A, Jelling I, et al. Acta Med Scand. 1987; 221: 165-70.

88. Wang YM, van Eys J. Annu Rev Nutr. 1981; 1: 437-75.

89. Wellhoener P, Fruehwald-Schultes B, Kern W, et al. J Clin Endocrinol Metab. 2000; 85: 1267-71.

90. Zakim D, Pardini RS, Herman RH, et al. Biochim Biophys Acta. 1967; 144: 242-51.

91. Zavaroni I, Sander S, Scott S, et al. Metabolism. 1980; 29: 970-3.

92. Zawalich WS, Rognstad R, Pagliara AS, et al. J Biol Chem. 1977; 252: 8519-23.

93. Zunft HJ, Schulze J, Gartner H, et al. Ann Nutr Metab. 1983; 27: 470-6.

Q

1. Bougoulia M, Tzotzas T, Efthymiou H, et al. Int J Obes Relat Metab Disord. 1999; 23: 625-8.

2. De Palo C, Macor C, Sicolo N, et al. Acta Diabetol Lat. 1989; 26: 155-62.

3. Evans K, Clark ML, Frayn KN. Clin Sci (Lond). 2001; 100: 493-8.

4. Glick Z, Wickler SJ, Stern JS, et al. J Nutr. 1984; 114: 1934-9.

5. Holt S, Brand J, Soveny C, et al. Appetite. 1992; 18: 129-41.

6. Jenkins AB, Markovic TP, Fleury A, et al. Diabetologia. 1997; 40: 348-51.

7. Marques-Lopes I, Forga L, Martinez JA. Nutrition. 2003; 19: 25-9.

8. Monteleone P, Bencivenga R, Longobardi N, et al. J Clin Endocrinol Metab. 2003; 88: 5510-4.

9. Muscelli E, Camastra S, Masoni A, et al. Eur J Clin Invest. 1996; 26: 940-3.

10. Raben A, Astrup A. Int J Obes Relat Metab Disord. 2000; 24: 450-9.

11. Romon M, Lebel P, Fruchart JC, et al. J Am Coll Nutr. 2003; 22: 247-51.

12. Romon M, Lebel P, Velly C, et al. Am J Physiol. 1999; 277(5 Pt 1): E855-61.

13. Suga A, Hirano T, Kageyama H, et al. Am J Physiol Endocrinol Metab. 2000; 278: E677-83.

14. Swaminathan R, King RF, Holmfield J, et al. Am J Clin Nutr. 1985; 42: 177-81.

15. Tentolouris N, Tsigos C, Perea D, et al. Metabolism. 2003; 52. 1426-32.

16. Van Gaal L, Mertens I, Vansant G, et al. J Endocrinol Invest. 1999; 22: 109-14.

Nutrition Labels

A

1. Guevin N, Jacques H, Nadeau A, et al. J Am Coll Nutr. 1996; 15: 389-96.

2. Ide T, Horii M, Yamamoto T, et al. Lipids. 1990; 25: 335-40.

3. Marlett JA, McBurney MI, Slavin JL; American Dietetic Association. J Am Diet Assoc. 2002; 102: 993-1000.

4. Nelson RW, Duesberg CA, Ford SL, et al. J Am Vet Med Assoc. 1998; 212: 380-6.

5. Okazaki H, Nishimune T, Matsuzaki H, et al. Int J Cancer. 2002; 100: 388-94.

6. Sunvold GD, Titgemeyer EC, Bourquin LD, et al. Am J Clin Nutr. 1995; 62: 1252-60.

7. Truswell AS. Curr Opin Lipidol. 1995; 6: 14-9.

8. Vuksan V, Korsic M, Posavi-Antonovic A. Lijec Vjesn. 1997; 119(3-4): 125-7.

9. Wolk A, Manson JE, Stampfer MJ, et al. JAMA. 1999; 281: 1998-2004.

Planning For The Future

A

1. Alfieri M, Pomerleau J, Grace DM. Obes Surg. 1997; 7: 9-15.

2. Alstrup KK, Gregersen S, Jensen HM, et al. Metabolism. 1999; 48: 22-9.

3. Bolton-Smith C, Woodward M. Int J Obes Relat Metab Disord. 1994; 18: 820-8.

4. Capito K, Hansen SE, Hedeskov CJ, et al. Acta Diabetol. 1992; 28(3-4): 193-8.

5. Elks ML. Cell Mol Biol. 1994; 40: 761-8.

6. Elks ML. Endocrinology. 1993; 133: 208-14.

7. Gravena C, Mathias PC, Ashcroft SJ. J Endocrinol. 2002; 173: 73-80.

8. Gremlich S, Roduit R, Thorens B. J Biol Chem. 1997; 272: 3216-22.

9. Hays JH, DiSabatino A, Gorman RT, et al. Mayo Clin Proc. 2003; 78: 1331-6.

10. Holness MJ, Greenwood GK, Smith ND, et al. Endocrinology. 2003; 144: 3958-68.

11. Lovejoy JC, Smith SR, Champagne CM, et al. Diabetes Care. 2002; 25: 1283-8.

12. Macdiarmid JI, Vail A, Cade JE, et al. Int J Obes Relat Metab Disord. 1998; 22: 1053-61.

13. McGloin AF, Livingstone MB, Greene LC, et al. Int J Obes Relat Metab Disord. 2002; 26: 200-7.

14. Miller WC, Lindeman AK, Wallace J, et al. Am J Clin Nutr. 1990; 52: 426-30.

15. Miller WC, Niederpruem MG, Wallace JP, et al. J Am Diet Assoc. 1994; 94: 612-5.

16. Nelson LH, Tucker LA. J Am Diet Assoc. 1996; 96: 771-7.

17. Pareja A, Tinahones FJ, Soriguer FJ, et al. Diabetes Res Clin Pract. 1997; 38: 143-9.

18. Prewitt TE, Schmeisser D, Bowen PE, et al. Am J Clin Nutr. 1991; 54: 304-10.

19. Ramirez R, Lopez JM, Bedoya FJ, et al. Diabetes Res. 1990; 15: 179-83.

20. Tucker LA, Seljaas GT, Hager RL. J Am Diet Assoc. 1997; 97: 981-6.

21. Vessby B, Karlstrom B, Boberg M, et al. Diabet Med. 1992; 9: 126-33.

22. Westerterp KR, Verboeket-van de Venne WP, Westerterp-Plantenga MS, et al. Int J Obes Relat Metab Disord. 1996; 20: 1022-6.

23. Zhou YP, Grill V. J Clin Endocrinol Metab. 1995; 80: 1584-90.

24. Zhou YP, Grill VE. J Clin Invest. 1994; 93: 870-6.

25. Zhou YP, Ling ZC, Grill VE. Metabolism. 1996; 45: 981-6.

B

1. Abbasi F, McLaughlin T, Lamendola C, et al. Am J Cardiol. 2000; 85: 45-8.

2. Chen YD, Coulston AM, Zhou MY, et al. Diabetes Care. 1995; 18: 10-6.

3. Coulston AM, Hollenbeck CB, Swislocki AL, et al. Am J Med. 1987; 82: 213-20.

4. Coulston AM, Hollenbeck CB, Swislocki AL, et al. Diabetes Care. 1989; 12: 94-101.

5. Coulston AM, Liu GC, Reaven GM. Metabolism. 1983; 32: 52-6.

6. Dreon DM, Fernstrom HA, Williams PT, et al. Am J Clin Nutr. 1999; 69: 411-8.

7. Fuh MM, Lee MM, Jeng CY, et al. Am J Hypertens. 1990; 3: 527-32.

8. Fukita Y, Gott o AM, Unger RH. Diabetes. 1975; 24: 552-8.

9. Garg A, Grundy SM, Koffler M. Diabetes Care. 1992; 15: 1572-80.

10. Ginsberg H, Olefsky JM, Kimmerling G, et al. J Clin Endocrinol Metab. 1976; 42: 729-35.

11. Golay A, Eigenheer C, Morel Y, et al. Int J Obes Relat Metab Disord. 1996; 20: 1067-72.

12. Grundy SM. N Engl J Med. 1986; 314: 745-8.

13. Hagenfeldt L, Hellstrom K, Wahren J. Clin Sci Mol Med. 1975; 48: 247-57.

14. Harris WS, Connor WE, Inkeles SB, et al. Metabolism. 1984; 33: 1016-9.

15. Hudgins LC, Hellerstein MK, Seidman CE, et al. J Lipid Res. 2000; 41: 595-604.

16. Jacobs B, De Angelis-Schierbaum G, Egert S, et al. J Nutr. 2004; 134: 1400-5.

17. Jeppesen J, Schaaf P, Jones C, et al. Am J Clin Nutr. 1997; 66: 437.

18. Kasim-Karakas SE, Almario RU, Mueller WM, et al. Am J Clin Nutr. 2000; 71: 1439-47.

19. Koutsari C, Malkova D, Hardman AE. Metabolism. 2000; 49: 1150-5.

20. Krauss RM, Dreon DM. Am J Clin Nutr. 1995; 62: 478S-487S.

21. Liu B, He Y, Zhang R, et al. Hua Xi Yi Ke Da Xue Xue Bao. 1990; 21: 145-9.

22. Liu G, Coulston A, Hollenbeck C, et al. J Clin Endocrinol Metab. 1984; 59: 636-42.

23. Liu GC, Coulston AM, Reaven GM. Metabolism. 1983; 32: 750-3.

24. Marckmann P, Sandstrom B, Jespersen J. Am J Clin Nutr. 1994; 59: 935-9.

25. Marques-Lopes I, Ansorena D, Astiasaran I, et al. Am J Clin Nutr. 2001; 73: 253-61.

26. McLaughlin T, Abbasi F, Lamendola C, et al. J Clin Endocrinol Metab. 2000; 85: 3085-8.

27. Mohanlal N, Holman RR. Diabetes Care. 2004; 27: 89-94.

28. O'Brien T, Nguyen TT, Buithieu J, et al. J Clin Endocrinol Metab. 1993; 77: 1345-51.

29. Olefsky JM, Crapo P, Reaven GM. Am J Clin Nutr. 1976; 29: 535-9.

30. Parks EJ, Rutledge JC, Davis PA, et al. J Cardiopulm Rehabil. 2001; 21: 73-9.

31. Pelkman CL, Fishell VK, Maddox DH, et al. Am J Clin Nutr. 2004; 79: 204-12.

32. Poppitt SD, Keogh GF, Prentice AM, et al. Am J Clin Nutr. 2002; 75: 11-20.

33. Sanfelippo ML, Swenson RS, Reaven GM. Kidney Int. 1977; 11: 54-61.

34. Schaefer EJ, Lamon-Fava S, Spiegelman D, et al. Metabolism. 1995; 44: 749-56.

35. Ullmann D, Connor WE, Hatcher LF, et al. Arterioscler Thromb. 1991; 11: 1059-67.

C

1. Allen NE, Appleby PN, Davey GK, et al. Cancer Epidemiol Biomarkers Prev. 2002; 11: 1441-8.

2. Allen NE, Appleby PN, Davey GK, et al. Br J Cancer. 2000; 83: 95-7.

3. Bissoli L, Di Francesco V, Ballarin A, et al. Ann Nutr Metab. 2002; 46: 73-9.

4. Blum A, Lupovitch S, Khazim K, et al. Clin Cardiol. 2001; 24: 463-6.

5. den Heijer M, Koster T, Blom HJ, et al. N Engl J Med. 1996; 334: 759-62.

6. Donner MG, Klein GK, Mathes PB, et al. Metabolism. 1998; 47: 273-9.

7. Fernandez-Miranda C, Aranda JL, Gomez Gonzalez P, et al. Med Clin (Barc). 1999; 113: 407-10.

8. Fruchart JC, Nierman MC, Stroes ES, et al. Circulation. 2004; 109(23 Suppl 1): III15-9.

9. Gao W, Jiang N, Zhu G. Zhonghua Yi Xue Za Zhi. 1998; 78: 821-3.

10. Geisel J, Hennen B, Hubner U, et al. Clin Chem Lab Med. 2003; 41: 1513-7.

11. Herrmann W, Geisel J. Clin Chim Acta. 2002; 326(1-2): 47-59.

12. Herrmann W, Schorr H, Obeid R, et al. Am J Clin Nutr. 2003; 78: 131-6.

13. Herrmann W, Schorr H, Purschwitz K, et al. Clin Chem. 2001; 47: 1094-101.

14. Huang YC, Chang SJ, Chiu YT, et al. Eur J Nutr. 2003, 42. 84-90.

15. Hung CJ, Huang PC, Lu SC, et al. J Nutr. 2002; 132: 152-8.

16. Krajcovicova-Kudlackova M, Blazicek P, Babinska K, et al. Scand J Clin Lab Invest. 2000; 60: 657-64.

17. Krajcovicova-Kudlackova M, Blazicek P, Kopcova J, et al. Ann Nutr Metab. 2000; 44: 135-8.

18. Laraqui A, Bennouar N, Meggouh F, et al. Ann Biol Clin (Paris). 2002; 60: 549-57.

19. Mann NJ, Li D, Sinclair AJ, et al. Eur J Clin Nutr. 1999; 53: 895-9.

20. Mark L, Erdei F, Marki-Zay J, et al. Orv Hetil. 2001; 142: 1611-5.

21. McCarty MF. Med Hypotheses. 2001; 56: 220-4.

22. McCarty MF. Med Hypotheses. 2003; 61: 323-34.

23. McCarty MF. Med Hypotheses. 2003; 60: 784-92.

24. Mezzano D, Kosiel K, Martinez C, et al. Thromb Res. 2000; 100: 153-60.

25. Mezzano D, Munoz X, Martinez C, el al. Thromb Haemost. 1999; 81: 913-7.

26. Noguchi T. Br J Nutr. 2000; 84 Suppl 2: S241-4.

27. Obeid R, Geisel J, Schorr H, et al. Eur J Haematol. 2002; 69(5-6): 275-9.

28. Parnetti L, Caso V, Santucci A, et al. Neurol Sci. 2004; 25: 13-7.

29. Ridker PM, Shih J, Cook TJ, et al. Circulation. 2002; 105: 1776-9.

30. Ridker PM, Stampfer MJ, Rifai N. JAMA. 2001; 285: 2481-5.

31. Seman LJ, McNamara JR, Schaefer EJ. Curr Opin Cardiol. 1999; 14: 186-91.

32. Takenaka A, Oki N, Takahashi SI, et al. J Nutr. 2000; 130: 2910-4.

33. van Beynum IM, Smeitink JA, den Heijer M, el al. Circulation. 1999; 99: 2070 2.

34. van der Molen EF, Verbruggen B, Novakova I, et al. BJOG. 2000; 107: 785-91.

35. Waldmann A, Koschizke JW, Leitzmann C, et al. Public Health Nutr. 2004; 7: 467-72.

36. Welch GN, Loscalzo J. N Engl J Med. 1998; 338: 1042-50.

37. Yildirir A, Tokgozoglu SL, Haznedaroglu I, et al. Angiology. 2001; 52: 589-96.

What To Expect

A

1. Acheson KJ, Schutz Y, Bessard T, et al. Am J Clin Nutr. 1988; 48: 240-7.

2. Chan ST, Johnson AW, Moore MH, et al. Hum Nutr Clin Nutr. 1982; 36: 223-32.

3. Shetty PS, Prentice AM, Goldberg GR, et al. Am J Clin Nutr. 1994; 60: 534-43.

4. Snitker S, Larson DE, Tataranni PA, et al. Am J Clin Nutr. 1997; 65: 941-6.

5. Wirrell EC, Darwish HZ, Williams-Dyjur C, et al. J Child Neurol. 2002; 17: 179-82.

6. Yang MU, Van Itallie TB. J Clin Invest. 1976; 58: 722-30.

B

1. Blake WL, Clarke SD. J Nutr. 1990; 120: 1727-9.

2. Boll M, Weber LW, Stampfl A. Z Naturforsch C. 1996; 51(11-12): 859-69.

3. Carrozza G, Livrea G, Caponetti R, et al. J Nutr. 1979; 109: 162-70.

4. Chascione C, Elwyn DH, Davila M, et al. Am J Physiol. 1987; 253(6 Pt 1): E664-9.

5. Clarke SD, Armstrong MK, Jump DB. J Nutr. 1990; 120: 218-24.

6. Clarke SD, Armstrong MK, Jump DB. J Nutr. 1990; 120: 225-31.

7. Foufelle F, Perdereau D, Gouhot B, et al. Eur J Biochem. 1992; 208: 381-7.

8. Hill JO, Lin D, Yakubu F, et al. Int J Obes Relat Metab Disord. 1992; 16: 321-33.

9. Kim H, Choi S, Lee HJ, et al. J Biochem Mol Biol. 2003; 36: 258-64.

10. Morris KL, Namey TC, Zemel MB. J Nutr Biochem. 2003; 14: 32-9.

11. Schwarz JM, Neese RA, Turner S, et al. J Clin Invest. 1995; 96: 2735-43.

12. Shillabeer G, Hornford J, Forden JM, et al. J Lipid Res. 1990; 31: 623-31.

13. Shillabeer G, Hornford J, Forden JM, et al. J Lipid Res. 1992; 33: 31-9.

14. Wolf G. Nutr Rev. 1996; 54(4 Pt 1): 122-3.

C

1. Keckwick A, Pawan GL. Metabolism. 1957; 6: 447-60.

2. Wirrell EC, Darwish HZ, Williams-Dyjur C, et al. J Child Neurol. 2002; 17: 179-82.

D

1. Gjedde A, Crone C. Am J Physiol. 1975; 229: 1165-9.

2. Hasselbalch SG, Knudsen GM, Jakobsen J, et al. J Cereb Blood Flow Metab. 1994; 14: 125-31.

3. Hasselbalch SG, Knudsen GM, Jakobsen J, et al. Am J Physiol. 1995; 268(6 Pt 1): E1161-6.

E

1. Flatt JP. Diabetes Metab Rev. 1988; 4: 571-81.

2. Flatt JP. Ann N Y Acad Sci. 1987; 499: 104-23.

3. Flatt JP. Am J Clin Nutr. 1995; 62: 820-36.

4. Schrauwen P, van Marken Lichtenbelt WD, Saris WH, et al. Am J Clin Nutr. 1997; 66: 276-82.

F

1. Burke LM, Angus DJ, Cox GR, et al. J Appl Physiol. 2000; 89: 2413-21.

2. Cox DJ, Palmer TN. Biochem J. 1987; 245: 903-5.

3. Fery F, Plat L, Balasse EO. J Clin Endocrinol Metab. 1998; 83: 2810-6.

4. Fery F, Plat L, Balasse EO. Metabolism. 2003; 52: 94-101.

5. Fery F, Plat L, Balasse EO. Am J Physiol. 1999; 277(5 Pt 1): E815-23.

6. Holness MJ, Kraus A, Harris RA, et al. Diabetes. 2000; 49: 775-81.

7. Holness MJ, Schuster-Bruce MJ, Sugden MC. Biochem J. 1988; 254: 855-9.

8. Leiter LA, Marliss EB. Clin Invest Med. 1983; 6: 287-92.

9. Peters SJ, Harris RA, Wu P, et al. Am J Physiol Endocrinol Metab. 2001; 281: E1151-8.

10. Pilegaard H, Helge JW, Saltin B, et al. FASEB J. 200; 15: A417.

11. Pilegaard H, Saltin B, Neufer PD. Diabetes. 2003; 52: 657-62.

G

1. Holness MJ, Kraus A, Harris RA, et al. Diabetes. 2000; 49: 775-81.

2. Peters SJ, Harris RA, Wu P, et al. Am J Physiol Endocrinol Metab. 2001; 281: E1151-8.

3. Pilegaard H, Helge JW, Saltin B, et al. FASEB J. 200; 15: A417.

Final Touches

A

1. Acheson KJ, Gremaud G, Meirim I, et al. Am J Clin Nutr. 2004; 79: 40-6.

2. Acheson KJ, Zahorska-Markiewicz B, Pittet P, et al. Am J Clin Nutr. 1980; 33: 989-97.

3. al'Absi M, Lovallo WR, McKey B, et al. Psychosom Med. 1998; 60: 521-7.

4. Ammaturo V, Monti M. Acta Med Scand. 1986; 220: 181-4.

5. Arciero PJ, Gardner AW, Calles-Escandon J, et al. Am J Physiol. 1995; 268(6 Pt 1): E1192-8.

6. Astrup A, Toubro S, Cannon S, et al. Am J Clin Nutr. 1990; 51: 759-67.

7. Battig K, Buzzi R, Martin JR, et al. Experientia. 1984; 40: 1218-23.

8. Baum D, French JW. Proc Soc Exp Biol Med. 1976; 151: 244-8.

9. Beaumont M, Batejat D, Pierard C, et al. J Sleep Res. 2001; 10: 265-76.

10. Bonnet MH, Arand DL. Physiol Behav. 1996; 59(4-5): 777-82.

11. Bonnet MH, Gomez S, Wirth O, et al. Sleep. 1995; 18: 97-104.

12. Bosqueiro JR, Carneiro EM, Bordin S, et al. Can J Physiol Pharmacol. 2000; 78: 462-8.

13. Bracco D, Ferrarra JM, Arnaud MJ, et al. Am J Physiol. 1995; 269(4 Pt 1): E671-8.

14. Brand-Miller J, Holt SH, de Jong V, et al. J Nutr. 2003; 133: 3149-52.

15. Brice CF, Smith AP. Psychopharmacology (Berl). 2002; 164: 188-92.

16. Bruce M, Scott N, Lader M, et al. Br J Clin Pharmacol. 1986; 22: 81-7.

17. Bruton JD, Lemmens R, Shi CL, et al. FASEB J. 2003; 17: 301-3.

18. Bryant CA, Farmer A, Tiplady B, et al. Eur J Clin Pharmacol. 1998; 54: 309-13.

19. Burns TW, Terry BE, Langley PE, et al. Diabetes. 1979; 28: 957-61.

20. Collins LC, Cornelius MF, Vogel RL, et al. Int J Obes Relat Metab Disord. 1994; 18: 551-6.

21. Costill DL, Dalsky GP, Fink WJ. Med Sci Sports. 1978; 10: 155-8.

22. Czok G. Z Ernahrungswiss. 1976; 15: 109-12.

23. De Matteis R, Arch JR, Petroni ML, et al. Int J Obes Relat Metab Disord. 2002; 26: 1442-50.

24. De Valck E, Cluydts R. J Sleep Res. 2001; 10: 203-9.

25. Dominquez MC, Herrera E. Horm Metab Res. 1976; 8: 33-7.

26. Dulloo AG, Duret C, Rohrer D, et al. Am J Clin Nutr. 1999; 70: 1040-5.

27. Dulloo AG, Geissler CA, Horton T, et al. Am J Clin Nutr. 1989; 49: 44-50.

28. Dyachok O, Gylfe E. J Biol Chem. 2004; 279: 45455-61.

29. Erickson MA, Schwarzkopf RJ, McKenzie RD. Med Sci Sports Exerc. 1987; 19: 579-83.

30. Fredholm BB. Pharmacol Toxicol. 1995; 76: 93-101.

31. Fukagawa NK, Veirs H, Langeloh G. Metabolism. 1995; 44: 630-8.

32. Goldrick RB, McLoughlin GM. J Clin Invest. 1970; 49: 1213-23.

33. Goldstein A, Kaizer S, Warren R. II. 1965; 150: 146-51.

34. Goldstein A, Wallace ME. Exp Clin Psychopharmacol. 1997; 5: 388-92.

35. Graham TE, Spriet LL. J Appl Physiol. 1991; 71: 2292-8.

36. Griffiths RR, Evans SM, Heishman SJ, et al. J Pharmacol Exp Ther. 1990; 252: 970-8.

37. Hagstrom-Toft E, Arner P, Johansson U, et al. Diabetologia. 1992; 35: 664-70.

38. Hetzler RK, Knowlton RG, Somani SM, et al. J Appl Physiol. 1990; 68: 44-7.

39. Hogervorst E, Riedel WJ, Kovacs E, et al. Int J Sports Med. 1999; 20: 354-61.

40. Holz GG, Leech CA, Heller RS, et al. J Biol Chem. 1999; 274: 14147-56.

41. Horne JA, Reyner LA. Psychophysiology. 1996; 33: 306-9.

The Carb Nite Solution

42. Islam MS, Leibiger I, Leibiger B, et al. Proc Natl Acad Sci U S A. 1998; 95: 6145-50.

43. Ivy JL, Costill DL, Fink WJ, et al. Med Sci Sports. 1979; 11: 6-11.

44. Izawa T, Koshimizu E, Komabayashi T, et al. Nippon Seirigaku Zasshi. 1983; 45: 36-44.

45. Izzo JL Jr, Ghosal A, Kwong T, et al. Am J Cardiol. 1983; 52: 769-73.

46. Jackman M, Wendling P, Friars D, et al. J Appl Physiol. 1996; 81: 1658-63.

47. James JE. Neuropsychobiology. 1998; 38: 32-41.

48. Jensen MD, Haymond MW, Gerich JE, et al. J Clin Invest. 1987; 79: 207-13.

49. Johnson LC, Spinweber CL, Gomez SA. Psychopharmacology (Berl). 1990; 101: 160-7.

50. Jung RT, Shetty PS, James WP, et al. Clin Sci (Lond). 1981; 60: 527-35.

51. Kamimori GH, Lugo SI, Penetar DM, et al. Int J Clin Pharmacol Ther. 1995; 33: 182-6.

52. Kamimori GH, Penetar DM, Headley DB, et al. Eur J Clin Pharmacol. 2000; 56: 537-44.

53. Kaplan GB, Greenblatt DJ, Ehrenberg BL, et al. J Clin Pharmacol. 1997; 37: 693-703.

54. Kelly TL, Mitler MM, Bonnet MH. Electroencephalogr Clin Neurophysiol. 1997; 102: 397-400.

55. Kenemans JL, Lorist MM. Pharmacol Biochem Behav. 1995; 52: 461-71.

56. Koot P, Deurenberg P. Ann Nutr Metab. 1995; 39: 135-42.

57. Kourtidou-Papadeli C, Papadelis C, Louizos AL, et al. Brain Res Cogn Brain Res. 2002; 13: 407-15.

58. Lachance MP, Marlowe C, Waddell WJ. Toxicol Appl Pharmacol. 1983; 71: 237-41.

59. Lagarde D, Batejat D, Sicard B, et al. Sleep. 2000; 23: 651-61.

60. Lane JD, Adcock RA, Williams RB, et al. Psychosom Med. 1990; 52: 320-36.

61. Laurent D, Schneider KE, Prusaczyk WK, et al. J Clin Endocrinol Metab. 2000; 85: 2170-5.

62. Leblanc J, Jobin M, Cote J, et al. J Appl Physiol. 1985; 59: 793–797.

63. Leblanc J, Richard D, Racotta IS. Pharmacol Res. 1995; 32: 129-33.

64. Lee MA, Flegel P, Cameron OG, et al. Psychiatry Res. 1988; 24: 61-5.

65. Lieberman HR, Wurtman RJ, Emde GG, et al. Psychopharmacology (Berl). 1987; 92: 308-12.

66. Liguori A, Grass JA, Hughes JR. Exp Clin Psychopharmacol. 1999; 7: 244-9.

67. Lovallo WR, Pincomb GA, Sung BH, et al. Hypertension. 1989; 14: 170-6.

68. Mohr T, Van Soeren M, Graham TE, et al. J Appl Physiol. 1998; 85: 979-85.

69. Mougios V, Ring S, Petridou A, et al. J Appl Physiol. 2003; 94: 476-84.

70. Muehlbach MJ, Walsh JK. Sleep. 1995; 18: 22-9.

71. Penetar D, McCann U, Thorne D, et al. Psychopharmacology (Berl). 1993; 112(2-3): 359-65.

72. Peters EJ, Klein S, Wolfe RR. Am J Physiol. 1991; 261(4 Pt 1): E500-4.

73. Petrie HJ, Chown SE, Belfie LM, et al. Am J Clin Nutr. 2004; 80: 22-8.

74. Pincomb GA, Lovallo WR, Passey RB, et al. Health Psychol. 1987; 6: 101-12.

75. Poehlman ET, LaChance P, Tremblay A, et al. Can J Physiol Pharmacol. 1989; 67: 10-6.

76. Potter JF, Haigh RA, Harper GD, et al. J Hum Hypertens. 1993; 7: 273-8.

77. Raguso CA, Coggan AR, Sidossis LS, et al. Metabolism. 1996; 45: 1153-60.

78. Ratzmann KP, Riemer D, Mannchen E, et al. Endokrinologie. 1976; 68: 319-26.

79. Reyner LA, Horne JA. Psychophysiology. 1997; 34: 721-5.

80. Robertson D, Frolich JC, Carr RK, et al. N Engl J Med. 1978; 298: 181-6.

81. Robertson D, Hollister AS, Kincaid D, et al. Am J Med. 1984; 77: 54-60.

82. Robertson D, Wade D, Workman R, et al. J Clin Invest. 1981; 67: 1111-7.

83. Ryu S, Choi SK, Joung SS, et al. J Nutr Sci Vitaminol (Tokyo). 2001; 47: 139-46.

84. Shepard JD, al'Absi M, Whitsett TL, et al. Am J Hypertens. 2000; 13(5 Pt 1): 475-81.

85. Silverman K, Mumford GK, Griffiths RR. Psychopharmacology (Berl). 1994; 114: 424-32.

86. Singh SP, Patel DG, Snyder AK, et al. Experientia. 1986; 42: 58-60.

87. Smith A, Thomas M, Perry K, et al. J Psychopharmacol. 1997; 11: 319-24.

88. Smits P, Pieters G, Thien T. Clin Pharmacol Ther. 1986; 40: 431-7.

89. Squires PE, Hills CE, Rogers GJ, et al. Eur J Pharmacol. 2004; 501(1-3): 31-39.

90. Sung BH, Lovallo WR, Pincomb GA, et al. Am J Cardiol. 1990; 65: 909-13.

91. Tanaka H, Nakazawa K, Arima M, et al. Brain Dev. 1984; 6: 355-61.

92. Thong FS, Graham TE. J Appl Physiol. 2002; 92: 2347-52.

93. Van Dongen HP, Price NJ, Mullington JM, et al. Sleep. 2001; 24: 813-9.

94. Van Soeren M, Mohr T, Kjaer M, et al. J Appl Physiol. 1996; 80: 999-1005.

95. Van Soeren MH, Graham TE. J Appl Physiol. 1998; 85: 1493-501.

96. Varadi A, Rutter GA. Diabetes. 2002; 51 Suppl 1: S190-201.

97. Walsh JK, Muehlbach MJ, Humm TM, et al. Psychopharmacology (Berl). 1990; 101: 271-3.

98. Waters WF, Magill RA, Bray GA, et al. Nutr Neurosci. 2003; 6: 221-35.

99. Wesensten NJ, Belenky G, Kautz MA, et al. Psychopharmacology (Berl). 2002; 159: 238-47.

100. Wesensten NJ, Belenky G, Thorne DR, et al. Aviat Space Environ Med. 2004; 75: 520-5.

101. Wright KP Jr, Badia P, Myers BL, et al. J Sleep Res. 1997; 6: 26-35.

102. Yoshida T, Sakane N, Umekawa T, et al. Int J Obes Relat Metab Disord. 1994; 18: 345-50.

103. Yoshioka K, Yoshida T, Kamanaru K, et al. J Nutr Sci Vitaminol (Tokyo). 1990; 36: 173-8.

104. Zahorska-Markiewicz B. Acta Physiol Pol. 1980; 31: 17-20.

105. Zhuravleva GN. Med Tr Prom Ekol. 1995; (2): 25-8.

B

1. Farshchi HR, Taylor MA, Macdonald IA. Eur J Clin Nutr. 2004; 58: 1071-7.

2. Farshchi HR, Taylor MA, Macdonald IA. Am J Clin Nutr. 2005; 81: 16-24.

C

1. Abramson EA, Arky RA. J Lab Clin Med. 1968; 72: 105-17.

2. Andreani D, Tamburrano G, Javicoli M. Horm Metab Res. 1976; Suppl 6: 99-105.

3. Avogaro A, Beltramello P, Gnudi L, et al. Diabetes. 1993; 42: 1626-34.

4. Ben G, Gnudi L, Maran A, et al. Am J Med. 1991; 90: 70-6.

5. Boden G, Chen X, DeSantis RA, et al. Am J Physiol. 1993; 265(2 Pt 1): E197-202.

6. Calderon-Attas P, Furnelle J, Christophe J. Biochim Biophys Acta. 1980; 620: 387-99.

7. Calissendorff J, Brismar K, Rojdmark S. Alcohol Alcohol. 2004; 39: 281-6.

8. Christiansen C, Thomsen C, Rasmussen O, et al. Eur J Clin Nutr. 1993; 47: 648-52.

9. Christiansen C, Thomsen C, Rasmussen O, et al. Br J Nutr. 1996; 76: 669-75.

10. Curtis-Prior PB. Experientia. 1972; 28: 1430-1.

11. Fielding BA, Reid G, Grady M, et al. Br J Nutr. 2000; 83: 597-604.

12. Fisher H, Halladay A, Ramasubramaniam N, et al. J Nutr. 2002; 132: 2732-6.

13. Hadley W, Koeslag JH, Lochner JD. Q J Exp Physiol. 1988; 73: 79-85.

14. Hansson P, Nilsson-Ehle P. Ann Nutr Metab. 1983; 27: 328-37.

15. Heikkonen E, Ylikahri R, Roine R, et al. Alcohol Clin Exp Res. 1998; 22: 437-43.

16. Kaffarnik H, Schneider J, Schubotz R, et al. Atherosclerosis. 1978; 29: 1-7.

17. Lang CH, Molina PE, Skrepnick N, et al. Am J Physiol. 1994; 266(6 Pt 1): E863-9.

18. Murgatroyd PR, Van De Ven ML, Goldberg GR, et al. Br J Nutr. 1996; 75: 33-45.

19. Nilsson NO, Belfrage P. J Lipid Res. 1978; 19: 737-411.

20. Nilsson-Ehle P. Lipids. 1978; 13: 433-7.

21. Raben A, Agerholm-Larsen L, Flint A, et al. Am J Clin Nutr. 2003; 77: 91-100.

22. Rojdmark S, Calissendorff J, Brismar K. Clin Endocrinol (Oxf). 2001; 55: 639-47.

23. Schubotz R, Muhlfellner G, Schneider J, et al. Res Exp Med (Berl). 1976; 167: 139-48.

24. Schutz Y. Proc Nutr Soc. 2000; 61: 319.

25. Shelmet JJ, Reichard GA, Skutches CL, et al. J Clin Invest. 1988; 81: 1137-45.

26. Sonko BJ, Prentice AM, Murgatroyd PR, et al. Am J Clin Nutr. 1994; 59: 619-25.

27. Suter PM, Schutz Y, Jequier E. N Engl J Med. 1992; 326: 983-7.

28. Teresinski G, Buszewicz G, Madro R. Forensic Sci Int. 2002; 127(1-2): 88-96.

29. Vexiau P, Legoff B, Cathelineau G. Horm Metab Res. 1983; 15: 419-21.

30. Wilson NM, Brown PM, Juul SM, et al. Br Med J (Clin Res Ed). 1981; 282: 849-53.

31. Wolfe BM, Havel JR, Marliss EB, et al. J Clin Invest. 1976; 57: 329-40.

D

1. Fernstrom JD. J Neural Transm Suppl. 1979; (15): 55-67.

2. Fernstrom JD. Appetite. 1988; 11 Suppl 1: 35-41.

3. Fernstrom JD, Wurtman RJ. Science. 1971; 174: 1023-5.

4. Lyons PM, Truswell AS. Am J Clin Nutr. 1988; 47: 433-9.

5. Rouch C, Meile MJ, Orosco M. Nutr Neurosci. 2003; 6: 117-24.

6. Spring B. Nutr Health. 1984; 3(1-2): 55-67.

7. Wurtman RJ, Wurtman JJ, Regan MM, et al. Am J Clin Nutr. 2003; 77: 128-32.

8. Yokogoshi H, Wurtman RJ. Metabolism. 1986; 35: 837-42.

9. Young SN. Can J Physiol Pharmacol. 1991; 69: 893-903.

E

1. Bennett FC, Ingram DM. Am J Clin Nutr. 1990; 52: 808-12.

2. Deutch B. Eur J Clin Nutr. 1995; 49: 508-16.

3. Johnson WG, Carr-Nangle RE, Bergeron KC. Psychosom Med. 1995; 57: 324-30.

4. Jones DY, Judd JT, Taylor PR, et al. Hum Nutr Clin Nutr. 1987; 41: 341-5.

5. Pedersen AB, Bartholomew MJ, Dolence LA, et al. Am J Clin Nutr. 1991; 53: 879-85.

6. Reichman ME, Judd JT, Taylor PR, et al. J Clin Endocrinol Metab. 1992; 74: 1171-5.

F

1. Belanger A, Locong A, Noel C, et al. J Steroid Biochem. 1989; 32: 829-33.

2. Clinton SK, Mulloy AL, Li SP, et al. J Nutr. 1997; 127: 225-237.

3. Dorgan JF, Judd JT, Longcope CH, et al. Am J Clin Nutr. 1997; 64: 850-855.

4. Goldin BR, Woods MN, Spiegelman DL, et al. Cancer. 1994; 74(3 Suppl): 1125-31.

5. Hamalainen E, Adlercreutz H, Puska P, et al. J Steroid Biochem. 1984; 20: 459-64.

6. Hanis T, Zidek V, Sachova J, et al. Br J Nutr. 1990; 61: 519-529.

7. Hill PB, Wynder EL. Cancer Lett. 1979; 7: 273-82.

8. Ingram DM, Bennett FC, Willcox D, et al. J Natl Cancer Inst. 1987; 79: 1225-9.

9. Key TJ, Roe L, Thorogood M, et al. Br J Nutr. 1990; 64: 111-9.

10. Perheentup A, Bergendahl M, Huhtaniemi I. Biol Reprod. 1995; 52: 808-813.

11. Raben A, Kiens B, Richter EA, et al. Med Sci Sports Exerc. 1992; 24: 1290-7.

12. Reed MJ, Cheng RW, Simmonds M, et al. J Clin Endocrinol Metab. 1987; 64: 1083-5.

13. Volek JS, Kraemer WJ, Bush JA, et al. J Appl Physiol. 1997; 82: 49-54.

G

1. El-Mallakh RS, Paskitti ME. Med Hypotheses. 2001; 57: 724-6.

H

1. Glick Z, Teague RJ, Bray GA. Science. 1981; 213: 1125-7.
2. Rigalleau V, Beylot M, Laville M, et al. Metabolism. 1999; 48: 278-84.
3. Rothwell NJ, Saville ME, Stock MJ. Am J Physiol. 1983; 245: E160-5.
4. Schwartz RS, Ravussin E, Massari M, et al. Metabolism. 1985; 34: 285 93.
5. Sidery MB, Gallen IW, Macdonald IA. Br J Nutr. 1990; 64: 705-13.

I

1. Rao SS, Kavelock R, Beaty J, et al. Gut. 2000; 46: 205-11.

Parting Words

A

1. Anti M, Armelao F, Marra G, et al. Gastroenterology. 1994; 107: 1709-18.
2. Anti M, Marra G, Armelao F, et al. Gastroenterology. 1992; 103: 883-91.
3. Augustsson K, Michaud DS, Rimm EB, et al. Cancer Epidemiol Biomarkers Prev. 2003; 12: 64-7.
4. Badawi AF, El-Sohemy A, Stephen LL, et al. Carcinogenesis. 1998; 19: 905-10.
5. Bagga D, Anders KH, Wang HJ, et al. Nutr Cancer. 2002; 42: 180-5.
6. Belzung F, Raclot T, Groscolas R. Am J Physiol. 1993; 264(6 Pt 2): R1111-8.
7. Berstad P, Seljeflot I, Veierod MB, et al. Clin Sci (Lond). 2003; 105: 13-20.
8. Boudreau MD, Sohn KH, Rhee SH, et al. Cancer Res. 2001; 61: 1386-91.
9. Braden LM, Carroll KK. Lipids. 1986; 21: 285-8.
10. Calder PC, Davis J, Yaqoob P, et al. Clin Sci (Lond). 1998; 94: 303-11.

11. Calder PC, Yaqoob P, Thies F, et al. Br J Nutr. 2002; 87 Suppl 1: S31-48.
12. Carroll KK, Hopkins GJ. Lipids. 1979; 14: 155-8.
13. Caygill CP, Charlett A, Hill MJ. Br J Cancer. 1996; 74: 159-64.
14. Chandrasekar B, Troyer DA, Venkatraman JT, et al. J Autoimmun. 1995; 8: 381-93.
15. Collie-Duguid ES, Wahle KW. Biochem Biophys Res Commun. 1996; 220: 969-74.
16. De Caterina R, Cybulsky MA, Clinton SK, et al. Prostaglandins Leukot Essent Fatty Acids. 1995; 52(2-3): 191-5.
17. De Caterina R, Cybulsky MI, Clinton SK, et al. Arterioscler Thromb. 1994; 14: 1829-36.
18. De Caterina R, Liao JK, Libby P. Am J Clin Nutr. 2000; 71(1 Suppl): 213S-23S.
19. De Caterina R, Libby P. Lipids. 1996; 31 Suppl: S57-63.
20. El-Sohemy A, Archer MC. Cancer Res. 1997; 57: 3685-7.
21. Fay MP, Freedman LS. Breast Cancer Res Treat. 1997; 46(2-3): 215-23.
22. Fay MP, Freedman LS, Clifford CK, et al. Cancer Res. 1997; 57: 3979-88.
23. Fernandes G. Nutr Rev. 1995; 53(4 Pt 2): S72-7; discussion S77-9.
24. Fickova M, Hubert P, Cremel G, et al. J Nutr. 1998; 128: 512-9.
25. Ge Y, Chen Z, Kang ZB, et al. Anticancer Res. 2002; 22(2A): 537-43.
26. Hilakivi-Clarke L, Clarke R, Onojafe I, et al. Proc Natl Acad Sci U S A. 1997; 94: 9372-7.
27. Hilakivi-Clarke L, Onojafe I, Raygada M, et al. J Natl Cancer Inst. 1996; 88: 1821-7.
28. Hursting SD, Thornquist M, Henderson MM. Prev Med. 1990; 19: 242-53.
29. Ide T, Kobayashi H, Ashakumary L, et al. Biochim Biophys Acta. 2000; 1485: 23-35.
30. Ide T, Murata M, Sugano M. J Lipid Res. 1996; 37: 448-63.
31. Iritani N, Komiya M, Fukuda H, et al. J Nutr. 1998; 128: 967-72.
32. James MJ, Cleland LG. Semin Arthritis Rheum. 1997; 27: 85-97.

33. Jolly CA, Muthukumar A, Avula CP, et al. J Nutr. 2001; 131: 2753-60.

34. Kaizer L, Boyd NF, Kriukov V, et al. Nutr Cancer. 1989; 12: 61-8.

35. Karmali RA, Marsh J, Fuchs C. J Natl Cancer Inst. 1984; 73: 457-61.

36. Kehn P, Fernandes G. J Clin Immunol. 2001; 21: 99-101.

37. Kikugawa K, Yasuhara Y, Ando K, et al. J Agric Food Chem. 2003; 51: 6073-9.

38. Kompauer I, Demmelmair H, Koletzko B, et al. Eur J Med Res. 2004; 9: 378-82.

39. Kromhout D. Med Oncol Tumor Pharmacother. 1990; 7(2-3): 173-6.

40. Kumamoto T, Ide T. Lipids. 1998; 33: 647-54.

41. Laidlaw M, Holub BJ. Am J Clin Nutr. 2003; 77: 37-42.

42. Larsson SC, Kumlin M, Ingelman-Sundberg M, et al. Am J Clin Nutr. 2004; 79: 935-45.

43. Leitzmann MF, Stampfer MJ, Michaud DS, et al. Am J Clin Nutr. 2004; 80: 204-16.

44. Lindner MA. Nutr Cancer. 1991; 15: 1-11.

45. Lopez-Garcia E, Schulze MB, Manson JE, et al. J Nutr. 2004; 134: 1806-11.

46. Lu S, Zhang X, Badawi AF, et al. Cancer Lett. 2002; 184: 7-12.

47. Madsen T, Skou HA, Hansen VE, et al. Am J Cardiol. 2001; 88: 1139-42.

48. Maillard V, Bougnoux P, Ferrari P, et al. Int J Cancer. 2002; 98: 78-83.

49. Mantzioris E, Cleland LG, Gibson RA, et al. Am J Clin Nutr. 2000; 72: 42-8.

50. Miles EA, Thies F, Wallace FA, et al. Clin Sci (Lond). 2001; 100: 91-100.

51. Narayanan BA, Narayanan NK, Reddy BS. Int J Oncol. 2001; 19: 1255-62.

52. Narisawa T, Takahashi M, Kotanagi H, et al. Jpn J Cancer Res. 1991; 82: 1089-96.

53. Norrish AE, Skeaff CM, Arribas GL, et al. Br J Cancer. 1999; 81: 1238-42.

54. Okita M, Yoshida S, Yamamoto J, et al. J Nutr Sci Vitaminol (Tokyo). 1995; 41: 313-23.

55. Okuno M, Kajiwara K, Imai S, et al. J Nutr. 1997; 127: 1752-7.

56. Okuyama H, Kobayashi T, Watanabe S. Prog Lipid Res. 1996; 35: 409-57.

57. Pietsch A, Weber C, Goretzki M, et al. Cell Biochem Funct. 1995; 13: 211-6.

58. Pischon T, Hankinson SE, Hotamisligil GS, et al. Circulation. 2003; 108: 155-60.

59. Raclot T, Groscolas R, Langin D, et al. J Lipid Res. 1997; 38: 1963-72.

60. Raheja BS, Sadikot SM, Phatak RB, et al. Ann N Y Acad Sci. 1993; 683: 258-71.

61. Rose DP, Connolly JM, Meschter CL. J Natl Cancer Inst. 1991; 83: 1491-5.

62. Sasaki S, Horacsek M, Kesteloot H. Prev Med. 1993; 22: 187-202.

63. Schmidt EB, Varming K, Pedersen JO, et al. Scand J Clin Lab Invest. 1992; 52: 229-36.

64. Simopoulos AP. Am J Clin Nutr. 1991; 54: 438-63.

65. Summers LK, Barnes SC, Fielding BA, et al. Am J Clin Nutr. 2000; 71: 1470-7.

66. Takahashi Y, Ide T. Br J Nutr. 2000; 84: 175-84.

67. Terry P, Lichtenstein P, Feychting M, et al. Lancet. 2001; 357: 1764-6.

68. Terry P, Wolk A, Vainio H, et al. Cancer Epidemiol Biomarkers Prev. 2002; 11: 143-5.

69. Tsai WS, Nagawa H, Kaizaki S, et al. J Gastroenterol. 1998; 33: 206-12.

70. Volker D, Fitzgerald P, Major G, et al. J Rheumatol. 2000; 27: 2343-6.

71. Wang H, Storlien LH, Huang XF. Am J Physiol Endocrinol Metab. 2002; 282: E1352-9.

72. Watkins BA, Li Y, Allen KG, et al. J Nutr. 2000; 130: 2274-84.

73. Wijendran V, Hayes KC. Annu Rev Nutr. 2004; 24: 597-615.

74. Wirfalt E, Mattisson I, Gullberg B, et al. Cancer Causes Control. 2002; 13: 883-93.

75. Yam D, Eliraz A, Berry EM. Isr J Med Sci. 1996; 32: 1134-43.

76. Yli-Jama P, Seljeflot I, Meyer HE, et al. Atherosclerosis. 2002; 164: 275-81.

B

1. Anderson JW, Story LJ, Zettwoch NC, et al. Diabetes Care. 1989; 12: 337-44.

2. Bray GA, Nielsen SJ, Popkin BM. Am J Clin Nutr. 2004; 79: 537-43.

3. Dwyer JT, Evans M, Stone EJ, et al. J Am Diet Assoc. 2001; 101: 798-802.

4. Elliott SS, Keim NL, Stern JS, et al. Am J Clin Nutr. 2002; 76: 911-22.

5. Farris RP, Nicklas TA, Myers L, et al. J Am Coll Nutr. 1998; 17: 579-85.

6. Guthrie JF, Morton JF. J Am Diet Assoc. 2000; 100: 43-51, quiz 49-50.

7. Kanarek RB, Orthen-Gambill N. J Nutr. 1982; 112: 1546-54.

8. Kasim-Karakas SE, Vriend H, Almario R, et al. J Lab Clin Med. 1996; 128: 208-13.

9. Kuczmarski RJ, Flegal KM, Campbell SM, et al. JAMA. 1994; 272: 205-11.

10. No authors listed. Pediatrics. 2004; 113(1 Pt 1): 152-4.

11. Rizkalla SW, Boillot J, Tricottet V, et al. Br J Nutr. 1993; 70: 199-209.

12. Schulze MB, Manson JE, Ludwig DS, et al. JAMA. 2004; 292: 927-934.

13. Sugawa-Katayama Y, Morita N. J Nutr. 1977; 107: 534-8.

14. Teff KL, Elliott SS, Tschop M, et al. J Clin Endocrinol Metab. 2004; 89: 2963-72.

C

1. Dansinger ML, Gleason JA, Griffith JL, et al. JAMA. 2005; 293: 43-53.

2. Foster GD, Wyatt HR, Hill JO, et al. N Engl J Med. 2003; 348: 2082-90.

D

1. Brehm BJ, Seeley RJ, Daniels SR, et al. J Clin Endocrinol Metab. 2003; 88: 1617-23.

2. Lewis SB, Wallin JD, Kane JP, et al. Am J Clin Nutr. 1977; 30: 160-70.

3. Rabast U, Kasper H, Schonborn J. Nutr Metab. 1978; 22: 269-77.

4. Samaha FF, Iqbal N, Seshadri P, et al. N Engl J Med. 2003; 348: 2074-81.

5. Sharman MJ, Gomez AL, Kraemer WJ, et al. J Nutr. 2004; 134: 880-5.

6. Sharman MJ, Volek JS. Clin Sci (Lond). 2004; 107: 365-9.

7. Stern L, Iqbal N, Seshadri P, et al. Ann Intern Med. 2004; 140: 778-85.

8. Volek JS, Sharman MJ, Gomez AL, et al. J Am Coll Nutr. 2004; 23: 177-84.

9. Westman EC, Yancy WS, Edman JS, et al. Am J Med. 2002; 113: 30-6.

10. Yancy WS Jr, Olsen MK, Guyton JR, et al. Ann Intern Med. 2004; 140: 769-77.

E

1. Chang NW, Huang PC. J Lipid Res. 1990; 31: 2141-7.

2. Doucet E, Almeras N, White MD, et al. Eur J Clin Nutr. 1998; 52: 2-6.

3. Garaulet M, Marin C, Perez-Llamas F, et al. J Physiol Biochem. 2004; 60: 39-49.

4. Gazzaniga JM, Burns TL. Am J Clin Nutr. 1993; 58: 21-8.

5. Lahoz C, Alonso R, Porres A, et al. Med Clin (Barc). 1999; 112: 133-7.

6. Merkel M, Velez-Carrasco W, Hudgins LC, et al. Proc Natl Acad Sci U S A. 2001; 98: 13294-9.

7. Navia B, Requejo AM, Ortega RM, et al. Ann Nutr Metab. 1997; 41: 299-306.

8. Nicklas TA, Hampl JS, Taylor CA, et al. Nutr Rev. 2004; 62: 132-41.

9. Salas J, Lopez Miranda J, Jansen S, et al. Med Clin (Barc). 1999; 114: 249.

F

1. Aarsland A, Chinkes D, Wolfe RR. Am J Clin Nutr. 1997; 65: 1774-82.

2. Acheson KJ, Schutz Y, Bessard T, et al. Am J Clin Nutr. 1988; 48: 240-7.

3. Alfieri M, Pomerleau J, Grace DM. Obes Surg. 1997; 7: 9-15.

4. Bobbioni-Harsch E, Habicht F, Lehmann T, et al. Eur J Clin Nutr. 1997; 51: 370-4.

5. Bolton-Smith C, Woodward M. Int J Obes Relat Metab Disord. 1994; 18: 820-8.

6. Dich J, Grunnet N, Lammert O, et al. Ugeskr Laeger. 2000; 162: 4794-9.

7. Hays JH, DiSabatino A, Gorman RT, et al. Mayo Clin Proc. 2003; 78: 1331-6.

8. Horton TJ, Drougas H, Brachey A, et al. Am J Clin Nutr. 1995; 62: 19-29.

The Carb Nite Solution

9. Lammert O, Grunnet N, Faber P, et al. Br J Nutr. 2000; 84: 233-45.

10. Macdiarmid JI, Vail A, Cade JE, et al. Int J Obes Relat Metab Disord. 1998; 22: 1053-61.

11. McDevitt RM, Bott SJ, Harding M, et al. Am J Clin Nutr. 2001; 74: 737-46.

12. McDevitt RM, Poppitt SD, Murgatroyd PR, et al. Am J Clin Nutr. 2000; 72: 369-77.

13. McGloin AF, Livingstone MB, Greene LC, et al. Int J Obes Relat Metab Disord. 2002; 26: 200-7.

14. Miller WC, Lindeman AK, Wallace J, et al. Am J Clin Nutr. 1990; 52: 426-30.

15. Miller WC, Niederpruem MG, Wallace JP, et al. J Am Diet Assoc. 1994; 94: 612-5.

16. Minehira K, Bettschart V, Vidal H, et al. Obes Res. 2003; 11: 1096-103.

17. Minehira K, Vega N, Vidal H, et al. Int J Obes Relat Metab Disord. 2004; 28: 1291-8.

18. Nelson LH, Tucker LA. J Am Diet Assoc. 1996; 96: 771-7.

19. Prewitt TE, Schmeisser D, Bowen PE, et al. Am J Clin Nutr. 1991; 54: 304-10.

20. Ravussin E, Schutz Y, Acheson KJ, et al. Am J Physiol. 1985; 249(5 Pt 1): E470-7.

21. Tucker LA, Seljaas GT, Hager RL. J Am Diet Assoc. 1997; 97: 981-6.

22. Welle SL, Campbell RG. Metabolism. 1983; 32: 889-93.

23. Westerterp KR, Verboeket-van de Venne WP, Westerterp-Plantenga MS, et al. Int J Obes Relat Metab Disord. 1996; 20: 1022-6.

24. Whitley HA, Humphreys SM, Samra JS, et al. Br J Nutr. 1997; 78: 15-26.

G

1. Nieman DC, Custer WF, Butterworth DE, et al. J Psychosom Res. 2000; 48: 23-9.

2. Racette SB, Schoeller DA, Kushner RF, et al. Am J Clin Nutr. 1995; 62: 345-9.

FAQs

A

1. Cunliffe A, Obeid OA, Powell-Tuck J. Eur J Clin Nutr. 1997; 51: 831-8.

2. Hirota N, Sone Y, Tokura H. J Physiol Anthropol Appl Human Sci. 2002; 21: 45-50.

3. Hurni M, Burnand B, Pittet P, et al. Br J Nutr. 1982; 47: 33-43.

4. Martin A, Normand S, Sothier M, et al. Br J Nutr. 2000; 84: 337-44.

B

1. Achten J, Gleeson M, Jeukendrup AE. Med Sci Sports Exerc. 2002; 34: 92-7.

2. Ahlborg G, Felig P, Hagenfeldt L, et al. J Clin Invest. 1974; 53: 1080-90.

3. Anderson RA, Polansky MM, Bryden NA, et al. Diabetes. 1982; 31: 212-6.

4. Bisschop PH, Sauerwein HP, Endert E, et al. Clin Endocrinol (Oxf). 2001; 54: 75-80.

5. Boyd AE 3rd, Giamber SR, Mager M, et al. Metabolism. 1974; 23: 531-42.

6. Duclos M, Corcuff JB, Arsac L, et al. Clin Endocrinol (Oxf). 1998; 48: 493-501.

7. Duclos M, Corcuff JB, Pehourcq F, et al. Eur J Endocrinol. 2001; 144: 363-8.

8. Duclos M, Corcuff JB, Rashedi M, et al. Eur J Appl Physiol. 1997; 75: 343-350.

9. Duclos M, Gouarne C, Bonnemaison D. J Appl Physiol. 2003; 94: 869-75.

10. Eliakim A, Brasel JA, Mohan S, et al. J Clin Endocrinol Metab. 1996; 81: 3986-92.

11. Essig DA, Alderson NL, Ferguson MA, et al. Metabolism. 2000; 49: 395-9.

12. Foricher JM, Ville N, Gratas-Delamarche A, et al. J Sports Med Phys Fitness. 2003; 43: 36-43.

13. Galbo H, Holst JJ, Christensen NJ. J Appl Physiol. 1975; 38: 70-6.

14. Galbo H, Holst JJ, Christensen NJ, et al. J Appl Physiol. 1976; 40: 855-63.

15. Gyntelberg F, Rennie MJ, Hickson RC, et al. J Appl Physiol. 1977; 43: 302-5.

16. Heitkamp HC, Schulz H, Rocker K, et al. Int J Sports Med. 1998; 19: 260-4.

17. Hirsch IB, Marker JC, Smith LJ, et al. Am J Physiol. 1991; 260(5 Pt 1): E695-704.

18. Hoogeveen AR, Zonderland ML. Int J Sports Med. 1996; 17: 423-8.

19. Jones NL, Heigenhauser GJ, Kuksis A, et al. Clin Sci (Lond). 1980; 59: 469-78.

20. Kanaley JA, Mottram CD, Scanlon PD, et al. J Appl Physiol. 1995; 79: 439-47.

21. Kanaley JA, Weatherup-Dentes MM, Alvarado CR, et al. Eur J Appl Physiol. 2001; 85(1-2): 68-73.

22. Kanaley JA, Weltman JY, Pieper KS, et al. J Clin Endocrinol Metab. 2001; 86: 2881-9.

23. Kang J, Hoffman JR, Wendell M, et al. Br J Sports Med. 2004; 38: 31-5.

24. Knechtle B, Muller G, Knecht H. Spinal Cord. 2004; 42: 564-72.

25. Knechtle B, Muller G, Willmann F, et al. Spinal Cord. 2004; 42: 24-8.

26. Lamarche B, Despres JP, Moorjani S, et al. Int J Obes Relat Metab Disord. 1993; 17: 255-61.

27. Lithell H, Hellsing K, Lundqvist G, et al. Acta Physiol Scand. 1979; 105: 312-5.

28. Luyckx AS, Pirnay F, Lefebvre PJ. Eur J Appl Physiol Occup Physiol. 1978, 39. 53-61.

29. Mertens DJ, Rhind S, Berkhoff F, et al. J Sports Med Phys Fitness. 1996; 36: 132-8.

30. Mora-Rodriguez R, Coyle EF. Am J Physiol Endocrinol Metab. 2000; 278: E669-76.

31. Phelain JF, Reinke E, Harris MA, et al. J Am Coll Nutr. 1997; 16: 140-6.

32. Roberts TJ, Weber JM, Hoppeler H, et al. J Exp Biol. 1996; 199 (Pt 8): 1651-8.

33. Romijn JA, Coyle EF, Sidossis LS, et al. Am J Physiol Endocrinol Metab. 1993; 265: E380-E391.

34. Satabin P, Bois-Joyeux B, Chanez M, et al. Eur J Appl Physiol Occup Physiol. 1989; 58: 583-90.

35. Seidman DS, Dolev E, Deuster PA, et al. Int J Sports Med. 1990; 11: 421-4.

36. Taskinen MR, Nikkila EA. Artery. 1980; 6: 471-83.

37. Thompson DL, Townsend KM, Boughey R, et al. Eur J Appl Physiol Occup Physiol. 1998; 78: 43-9.

38. Tuttle KR, Marker JC, Dalsky GP, et al. Am J Physiol. 1988; 254(6 Pt 1): E713-9.

39. Tyndall GL, Kobe RW, Houmard JA. Eur J Appl Physiol Occup Physiol. 1996; 73(1-2): 61-5.

40. van Loon LJ, Greenhaff PL, Constantin Teodosiu D, et al. J Physiol. 2001; 536(Pt 1): 295-304.

41. Vasankari TJ, Kujala UM, Heinonen OJ, et al. Acta Endocrinol (Copenh). 1993; 129: 109-13.

42. Weltman A, Weltman JY, Womack CJ, et al. Med Sci Sports Exerc. 1997; 29: 669-76.

43. Wesche MF, Wiersinga WM. Horm Metab Res. 2001; 33: 423-7.

44. Whitley HA, Humphreys SM, Campbell IT, et al. J Appl Physiol. 1998; 85: 418-24.

45. Winder WW, Hickson RC, Hagberg JM, et al. J Appl Physiol. 1979; 46: 766-71.

C

1. Schrauwen P, Lichtenbelt WD, Saris WH, et al. Am J Physiol. 1998; 274(6 Pt 1): E1027-33.

2. Schrauwen P, van Marken Lichtenbelt WD, Saris WH, et al. Am J Physiol. 1997; 273(3 Pt 1): E623-9.

3. Smith SR, de Jonge L, Zachwieja JJ, et al. Am J Clin Nutr. 2000; 72: 131-8.

4. Thomas CD, Peters JC, Reed GW, et al. Am J Clin Nutr. 1992; 55: 934-42.

D

1. Rigalleau V, Beylot M, Laville M, et al. Metabolism. 1999; 48: 278-84.

E

1. Fiebig R, Griffiths MA, Gore MT, et al. J Nutr. 1998; 128: 810-7.

2. Fukuda H, Iritani N, Tanaka T. J Nutr Sci Vitaminol (Tokyo). 1983; 29: 691-9.

3. Glick Z, Teague RJ, Bray GA. Science. 1981; 213: 1125-7.

4. Herzberg GR, Rogerson M. Br J Nutr. 1988; 59: 233-41.

The Carb Nite Solution

5. Rothwell NJ, Saville ME, Stock MJ. Am J Physiol. 1983; 245: E160-5.

F

1. Gill K, Amit Z. A review of recent studies. Recent Dev Alcohol.1989; 7: 225-48.

2. Koob GF, Roberts AJ, Schulteis G, et al. Alcohol Clin Exp Res. 1998; 22: 3-9.

3. Naranjo CA, Sellers EM. Recent Dev Alcohol. 1989; 7: 255-66.

4. Naranjo CA, Sellers EM, Lawrin MO. J Clin Psychiatry. 1986; 47 Suppl: 16-22.

5. Naranjo CA, Sellers EM, Sullivan JT, et al. Clin Pharmacol Ther. 1987; 41: 266-74.

6. Zabik JE. Recent Dev Alcohol. 1989; 7: 211-23.

G

1. Diener HC, Dethlefsen U, Dethlefsen-Gruber S, et al. Int J Clin Pract. 2002; 56: 243-6.

2. Fung MC, Holbrook JH. West J Med. 1989; 151: 42-4.

3. Jones K, Castleden CM. Age Ageing. 1983; 12: 155-8.

4. Man-Son-Hing M, Wells G. BMJ. 1995; 310: 13-7.

5. Mandal AK, Abernathy T, Nelluri SN, et al. J Clin Pharmacol. 1995; 35: 588-93.

6. Sidorov J. J Am Geriatr Soc. 1993; 41: 498-500.

H

1. Lin YC, Lyle RM, McCabe LD, et al. J Am Coll Nutr. 2000; 19: 754-60.

2. Melanson EL, Sharp TA, Schneider J, et al. Int J Obes Relat Metab Disord. 2003; 27: 196-203.

3. Papakonstantinou E, Flatt WP, Huth PJ, et al. Obes Res. 2003; 11: 387-94.

4. Shi H, Dirienzo D, Zemel MB. FASEB J. 2001; 15: 291-3.

5. Shi H, Halvorsen YD, Ellis PN, et al. Physiol Genomics. 2000; 3: 75-82.

6. Zemel MB, Shi H, Greer B, et al. FASEB J. 2000; 14: 1132-8.

7. Zemel MB, Thompson W, Milstead A, et al. Obes Res. 2004; 12: 582-90.

I

1. Gannon MC, Nuttall FQ, Lane JT, et al. Metabolism. 1992; 41: 1137-45.

2. Nuttall FQ, Gannon MC. Metabolism. 1990; 39: 749-55.

J

1. Alberts DS, Martinez ME, Roe DJ, et al. Phoenix Colon Cancer Prevention Physicians' Network. 2000; 342: 1156-62.

2. Bonithon-Kopp C, Kronborg O, Giacosa A, et al. European Cancer Prevention Organisation Study Group. 2000; 356: 1300-6.

3. Jacobs ET, Giuliano AR, Roe DJ, et al. J Natl Cancer Inst. 2002; 94: 1620-5.

4. Jacobs ET, Giuliano AR, Roe DJ, et al. Cancer Epidemiol Biomarkers Prev. 2002; 11: 1699.

5. Schatzkin A, Lanza E, Corle D, et al. Polyp Prevention Trial Study Group. 2000; 342: 1149-55.

K

1. Driver HS, Shulman I, Baker FC, et al. Physiol Behav. 1999; 68(1-2): 17-23.

2. Halberg F. J Nutr. 1989; 119: 333-43.

3. Hirsh E, Halberg F, Goetz FC, et al. Chronobiologia. 1975; 2(suppl 1): 31-32.

4. Jacobs H, Thompson M, Halberg E, et al. Chronobiologia. 1975; 2(suppl 1): 33.

5. Keim NL, Van Loan MD, Horn WF, et al. J Nutr. 1997; 127: 75-82.

6. Nelson W, Halberg F. J Nutr. 1986; 116: 2244-53.

7. Nelson W, Scheving L, Halberg F. J Nutr. 1975; 105: 171-84.

8. Philippens KM, von Mayersbach H, Scheving LE. J Nutr. 1977; 107: 176-93.

9. Sensi S, Capani F. Chronobiol Int. 1987; 4: 251-61.

10. Zammit GK, Ackerman SH, Shindledecker R, et al. Physiol Behav. 1992; 52: 251-9.

L

1. Foster GD, Wyatt HR, Hill JO, et al. N Engl J Med. 2003; 348: 2082-90.

M

1. Brooks SP, Lampi BJ. Comp Biochem Physiol B Biochem Mol Biol. 1997; 118: 359-65.

N

1. De Lorenzo A, Petrone-De Luca P, Sasso GF, et al. Respiration. 1999; 66: 407-12.
2. Despres JP, Bouchard C, Tremblay A, et al. Med Sci Sports Exerc. 1985; 17: 113-8.
3. Douchi T, Yamamoto S, Oki T, et al. Maturitas. 2000; 35: 25-30.
4. Jones PR, Edwards DA. Ann Hum Biol. 1999; 26: 151-62.
5. Kohrt WM, Obert KA, Holloszy JO. J Gerontol. 1992; 47: M99-105.
6. Mayo MJ, Grantham JR, Balasekaran G. Med Sci Sports Exerc. 2003; 35: 207-13.
7. Nindl BC, Friedl KE, Marchitelli LJ, et al. Med Sci Sports Exerc. 1996; 28: 786-93.

8. Nindl BC, Harman EA, Marx JO, et al. J Appl Physiol. 2000; 88: 2251-9.
9. Rebuffe-Scrive M, Lonnroth P, Marin P, et al. Int J Obes. 1987; 11: 347-55.
10. Treuth MS, Ryan AS, Pratley RE, et al. J Appl Physiol. 1994; 77: 614-20.
11. Weinsier RL, Hunter GR, Gower BA, el al. Am J Clin Nutr. 2001; 74: 631-6.

O

1. Hemingway C, Freeman JM, Pillas DJ, et al. Pediatrics. 2001; 108: 898-905.
2. Liu YM, Williams S, Basualdo-Hammond C, et al. J Am Diet Assoc. 2003; 103: 707-12.

P

1. Colombo P, Mangano M, Bianchi PA, et al. Scand J Gastroenterol. 2002; 37: 3-5.
2. Iwakiri K, Kobayashi M, Kotoyori M, et al. Dig Dis Sci. 1996; 41: 926-30.
3. Pehl C, Pfeiffer A, Waizenhoefer A, et al. Aliment Pharmacol Ther. 2001; 15: 233-9.
4. Pehl C, Waizenhoefer A, Wendl B, et al. Am J Gastroenterol. 1999; 94: 1192-6.
5. Penagini R. Eur J Gastroenterol Hepatol. 2000; 12: 1343-5.
6. Penagini R, Mangano M, Bianchi PA. Gut. 1998; 42: 330-3.

Index

Made in the USA
San Bernardino, CA
06 April 2014